Tán

女醫雜言

Miscellaneous Records of a Female Doctor

Nǔ Yī Zá Yán

Lorraine Wilcox, L.Ac.
Dr. Yue Lu, L.Ac., Dipl.Ac.

The Chinese Medicine Database
www.cm-db.com
Portland, Oregon

Miscellaneous Records of a Female Doctor

女醫雜言

Nǔ Yī Zá Yán

Lorraine Wilcox
Yue Lu

Copyright © 2015 The Chinese Medicine Database

1017 SW Morrison #306
Portland, OR 97205 USA

COMP designation original Chinese work and English translation

Cover Design by Jonathan Schell L.Ac.
Library of Congress Cataloging-in-Publication Data:

Tán Yǔnxián, fl. 1461 - 1554
 [Miscellaneous Records of a Female Doctor. English]
 Nü Yi Za Yan = Miscellaneous Records of a Female Doctor.
 / translation Lorraine Wilcox
  p. cm.
 Includes Index.
 ISBN 978-0-9906029-0-3 (alk. paper)
 Medicine, Chinese   I. Wilcox, Lorraine. II. Title: Miscellaneous
 Records of a Female Doctor.

International Standard Book Number (ISBN): 978-0-9906029-0-3
Printed in the United States of America

Contents

Appendices

Indices

Dedication:
For all the ancient female doctors whose names we will never know.

Forward by Charlotte Furth

It is a great pleasure to have Tán Yǔnxián get full-length book treatment, and to see this done by Lorraine Wilcox, who like her subject combines the skills of practitioner and scholar. I was privileged to be in the pioneer generation of Westerners who discovered so many treasures of Chinese medical history in the 1980s, and to count Lorraine Wilcox as a friend from the world of Chinese medical education in contemporary Los Angeles. Now she offers us a more complete look at the rare textual legacy of this *Míng* dynasty woman practitioner.

Using a recently discovered additional printed edition and its prefaces, she provides as full a biography as we are likely to find. Using now abundant digital resources, she has scrupulously excavated an authoritative text for her translation. Most impressive for us pure scholars of Chinese medical history, she has presented Tán Yǔnxián's prescriptions in detail. We see not only the exact ingredients, but also the many sources she drew upon from the *Sòng-Yuán* medical masters; and how the methods of preparation she recommended link pharmacy to domestic culinary arts.

As an accomplished practitioner herself, Wilcox uses prescriptions to better explain how each case manifests the illness syndromes of Chinese medicine. Where relevant she suggests biomedical comparisons. She wants Tán Yǔnxián to stand in for the countless women doctors who will forever remain unknown, and for her medical learning to be a resource for practitioners today.

I am very pleased that my friend Lorraine has asked me to write an introduction to this fine piece of work.

Charlotte Furth
Professor Emerita of Chinese History, University of Southern California

Translator's Introduction to
Nǚ Yī Zá Yán《 女醫雜言 》(Miscellaneous Records of a Female Doctor) by Tán Yǔnxián 談允賢

Tán Yǔnxián's Life

Tán Yǔnxián was the author of this book of case studies entitled *Miscellaneous Records of a Female Doctor*. She was from the city of Wúxī in Jiāngsū Province (江蘇無錫), near to Sūzhōu and not far from Shànghǎi. Tán was born about 1461 and died around 1556 (mid-*Míng* dynasty).[1]

The Tán family was made up of scholars and scholarly doctors, not uncommon at the time. Her paternal Grandfather Tán and Grandmother Rú (Chinese women did not change their names when they married) were both doctors, although the grandfather also gained official rank. Fortunately for Tán, none of the males in her father's or her own generation wanted to become a doctor. Tán was a bright child, so her grandparents decided to teach her medicine and pass down their skills.

Tán's main teacher was her grandmother. This was probably due to the pre-scribed manner in which males and females, even of the same family, were to interact. But it is likely that the grandmother specialized in the treatment of women and recognized that Tán's patients would be women too. Tán memo-rized medical books, asked questions of her grandparents, and perhaps helped them in clinic.

---

1. These dates are based on Tán mentioning (in her preface to the 1511 edition) that she was 50 years old when she published her book and her grand-nephew stating (in a postscript to the 1585 edition) that she was 96 when she died. It is possible that these dates are not precise as Tán may have rounded off her age to 50.

Tán married at about the age of 15 (as was standard at the time) and went to live with her husband's family, surnamed Yáng. It must have been in the same city since she described continued contact with her grandmother. After this, Tán concentrated on raising her one son and three daughters. As a young mother, she did not report having patients except her own children when they became ill. She treated them, supervised by Grandmother Rú. Later, Grandmother Rú became ill and passed her medical books and materials on to Tán. After the grandmother died, Tán also fell seriously ill until Grandmother Rú visited her in a dream and told her where to find the cure.

At that point it seems that Tán found her power. She began treating women and became popular as a doctor. One might be tempted to say she specialized in female diseases, but this is only a partial truth. Tán specialized in female patients, treating most any disorder a women might have. Interaction between the genders was highly restricted and women strongly preferred to see a female doctor if they could. Besides menstruation, fertility, pregnancy, and postpartum diseases, Tán treated insomnia, pain, skin problems, fevers, and so forth. She treated girls as well as women, although none of her cases in the book involved infants.

At the time, women of high ranking families did not deal with affairs outside of their household, so at the age of fifty, Tán asked her son to publish these thirty-one medical cases. Tán's own preface tells her story up until this point. We do not know if she continued writing after the book was published, but no later writings survive.

Tán's later years were filled with sorrow. In a postscript to the 1585 edition, Tán's grand-nephew described the tragedies that befell her son and grandson. Since Tán lived to the age of 96, she was probably was alive when they died. The grand-nephew republished *Miscellaneous Records* as an act of filial piety, but he had a hard time finding even one copy to work from. He didn't even know his great-aunt had written a book until he came across a draft of his grandfather's preface to it. The grand-nephew did, however, remember seeing Tán treat patients when he was a child.

Tangentially, it seems Tán's grandfather, named Tán Fù, also wrote a book called *Xiān Chuán Yì Fang* (Unusual Formulas Passed Down by an Immortal).[2] It is not known whether this book was originally printed or hand copied, but in 1602 Tán's same grand-nephew[3] also had it published by the same company (*Chún Jìng Táng* 純敬堂) that reprinted Miscellaneous Records. It is said to include fifteen secret family formulas and has a large number of illustrations.[4]

Nǚ Yī Zá Yán (Miscellaneous Records of a Female Doctor) has two sets of stories in it. Tán's life story is told in the prefaces and postscripts. Then glimpses of the lives Tán's patients are seen in the cases. Some may read this book only for the medicine, but I found these stories moving and I hope the reader will too.

Timeline for Tán Yǔnxián and
Miscellaneous Records of a Female Doctor

1461	Tán was born.
1492	Her younger brother was a successful candidate in the examinations as a scholar (not a doctor).
1510	Tán wrote the preface to her book.
1511	First edition published by her son when Tán was 50 years old. No known copies of this edition survive.
1556	Tán died (96 years old).
1585	Second edition (woodblock print, *Chún Jìng Táng* publishing company) published by her great-nephew Tán Xiū to honor her branch of the family since Tán had no living descendants. He had a hard time finding a copy, so the book was almost lost at this time.
1999	Charlotte Furth published *A Flourishing Yin*, which contains about ten pages describing this book. She obtained photos

---

2. 談復《仙傳異方》.
3. Tán Fù was the great-great-grandfather of Tán's grand-nephew.
4. This book came up in a search, appearing on an auction site from 2013, but no copies are currently available.

of the one surviving 1585 woodblock print edition from the rare book library of the Beijing Institute of Traditional Chinese Medicine.

2007   The Traditional Chinese Medicine Classics Press[5] printed two hundred copies of a photocopy of the same surviving 1585 edition. It seems impossible to find any of these 200 copies except through libraries that collect such things.

2015   This edition with English translation was published by The Chinese Medicine Database.

Many ancient medical books have been reprinted in Chinese and many have electronic versions readily available on the internet. But up until now, *Miscellaneous Records* cannot be found electronically or in print (except for the 200 copies mentioned above, but none are available for sale). *Miscellaneous Records* has almost been lost two or three times. My hope is that now Tán Yǔnxián will remembered and *Miscellaneous Records of a Female Doctor* will not be lost again.

About the Text

Miscellaneous Records of a Female Doctor is the earliest known writings by a female doctor in China. It consists of one volume with 31 cases surrounded by two prefaces and three postscripts. Counting all this (but not the title pages and so forth), the 1585 edition was only 51 pages.

One of the two prefaces was written by Tán herself and tells her story up until the time the book was published. One of the prefaces and one of the postscripts were written by high ranking officials related to Tán. Another postscript was written by her younger brother, also in the government service. The thirty-one cases and these prefaces and postscripts were present in the 1511 edition. The 1585 edition also contains a postscript by Tán's grand-nephew (the grandson of her younger brother). This postscript describes Tán's later years, the fate of her descendants, and the story of how the book was republished. It

---

5. Zhōngyī gǔjí chūbǎn shè 中醫古籍出版社, Běijīng.

also mentioned that the printing plates for some other prefaces or postscripts were lost, so these were not reprinted.

The body of the book consists of the thirty-one cases. There is no general discussion of medicine or the treatment of disease, no overview of her practice or her patients. The cases stand alone. See below for further discussion of their content.

The title of the book is *Miscellaneous Records of a Female Doctor*. More literally *zá yán* 雜言 would be translated as *miscellaneous words*. Others have translated it as *miscellaneous sayings*, but this is not a collection of sayings; it is thirty-one cases and nothing else. While *yán* 言 means words, speech, or talk, I took the liberty to change it to *records*. *Zá* 雜 means miscellaneous, mixed, or even confused. In this context, however, its opposite can be seen as *lèi* 類 which can mean categorized. This is a book with cases in more or less random order, not organized by category so perhaps we could call it *Uncategorized Cases of a Female Doctor*. The order of the cases does not follow any strict plan, unless they are organized by date (they are not individually dated). They were not arranged by disease like many of the later and larger case study books.

In addition, the title of the book has a casual feel for the Chinese reader, as if Tán were not taking herself too seriously. In fact, all of her writing uses very humble terms for herself and her achievements, unlike many of her male contemporaries. Was this because she felt her achievements were small? Was this because proper etiquette for a woman was to be extremely humble and this had become second nature to Tán? Was this a strategy to avoid ruffling the feathers of the men who might read it and think she was too uppity? We cannot know.

Methodology for the Translator's Comments

I trained first as a practitioner of Chinese medicine. After becoming licensed, I grew more and more interested in the roots of the medicine and the older ways of practicing. I informally studied Chinese language, especially the language of the old medical texts, and began translating for my own knowledge and pleasure. I have always tended to be more interested in books published by university presses than books written for practitioners. One could say I am a practitioner with scholarly tendencies, but I am not a formally trained scholar of the history of Chinese medicine or classical Chinese language. My translations are written for practitioners who also want to understand the concepts contained in the old books. True academics will not be satisfied with my work; neither will practitioners who only want to know how to treat various conditions. I function at the cusp. That being said, here is how I did the research for my commentary.

Tán most often named a formula and the source book where she found it. Then she mentioned any modifications; however she did not include the details for the formula itself such as the ingredients, their doses, and so forth. She expected her readers to be familiar with the formulas and to have access to the same sources. Unfortunately, this is not the case today. Some of the books she named have been lost (meaning there are no known existing copies); some of them may be available only in a rare books collection in China, but the translator lacks access. Sometimes Tán named a formula and a source book, but there is no formula by that name in the book. Did she have a different edition of the book? Was it there under a different name? Was she mistaken about the source?

The good news is that many of her formulas are still commonly used today. Even for those that are not, quite a few of the source books still exist and are available. In these cases, I translated the formula from the source she mentioned and included this in the commentary.[6]

Tán attributed many of her formulas to "*Dān Xī Fāng* 《 丹溪方 》" literally "Zhū Dānxī's Formulas." Was this the name of a particular book? If so, there is no mention of it elsewhere. It is likely this meant it was a formula in a book attributed to Zhū Dānxī or one of his close disciples. Or perhaps her family had a book in which someone had compiled many of Zhū's formulas. In any case,

---

6. The Chinese characters are included for all of Tán's writings, but not for translations of formulas in my commentary. However, the formulas in the commentary are translated from ancient sources and the name of the source is cited.

I looked for formulas attributed to '*Dān Xī Fāng*' in the books written by Zhū Dānxī or his followers, especially in *Dān Xī Zhì Fǎ Xīn Yào* and *Dān Xī Xīn Fǎ*.[7]

Zhū, who had lived about 200 years earlier than Tán, was from a neighboring province and his works were quite popular. English-speaking people are most aware that Zhū was one of the four great masters of the *Jīn-Yuán* period and the founder of the school of nourishing yīn. In fact, while he did develop this theory, Zhū treated all kinds of conditions, many of them unrelated to depletion of yīn. His books contain practical information and formulas for treating a wide spectrum of conditions. Tán did not seem to subscribe to a specific theoretical school of thought; she simply found his formulas effective.

When available, I translated a formula from the named source. When the source book was unavailable or when a formula could not be found in the named source, I had to become a medical detective.

- First I checked books I knew Tán used for other formulas.
- Then I checked various Zhū Dānxī-related sources, since Tán was fond of his formulas.
- If these failed I looked for sources published before the sixteenth century because these books would be known during Tán's life.
- Finally, if no source could be found that pre-dated Tán, I looked for later formulas, but keeping them as close as possible in time. Many formulas were passed down in book after book. When an earlier source is lost, the same formula is often found in a later book.
- Sometimes multiple formulas with the same name were discovered. In this case I selected the most likely candidate(s) based on the above criteria as well as looking for the one that best matched the condition being treated. On occasion I gave two possibilities in my commentary.

In all cases, the recipe given in my commentary comes directly from an ancient source.

Beyond this, I wrote about the nature or etiology of the disease, and tried to explain anything else that might be unfamiliar or seem odd to the modern reader.

7. Please see the book appendix for details on various books mentioned in the text or commentary.

13

If your interest is not in the practice of medicine, but is instead in the lives of women in *Míng* China, by all means skip over the more technical commentary on the formulas and diseases.

The History of Medical Case Studies

The medical case history is a particular form of writing that developed over the course of time. Many ancient history books contained them. Often they were just a story that involved disease but they were not written to aid the learning of doctors. An example of this type is the story is found in *Zuǒ Zhuàn*[8] regarding the Duke of Jìn who had a disease hiding in the *gāo-huāng*.

The most famous cases in ancient history books are found in Volume 105 of the Historical Records (*Shǐ Jì*) by Sīmǎ Qiān (*Hàn*)[9] which describes the story of Biǎn Què 扁鵲 and twenty-five cases of Chúnyú Yì 淳于意 (2nd c. BCE). These twenty-five cases were presented by Chúnyú Yì as his defense in a court case.[10] When read, the medical language feels familiar, yet it is still quite different from the medicine that came after *Nèi Jīng*.

---

8. 《左傳》. Here is the story as retold in *Zhēn Jiǔ Dà Chéng*:
《左傳》成公十年，晉侯疾病，求醫於秦，秦使醫緩〔秦醫名緩〕為之，未至。公夢疾為二豎子，曰：彼良醫也，懼傷我，焉逃之？其一曰：居肓之上，膏之下，若我何？醫至曰：疾不可為也。在肓之上，膏之下，攻之不可，達之不及，藥不至焉，不可為也？公曰：良醫也。厚為之禮而歸之。《針灸大成》
Zuǒ Zhuàn says: During the tenth year of Chéng Gōng, the Duke of Jìn took ill. He sought a physician in Qín. Qín employed Yī Huǎn to serve him. The doctor had not yet arrived when the duke dreamed of his disease as two boys, who said, "That is a good physician; I fear he will hurt us. How can we escape?" The other said, "What if we dwell above the *huāng* [diaphragm] and below the *gāo* [the region below the heart]?" The physician arrived and said, "The disease cannot be treated. It is located above the *huāng* and below the *gāo*. It cannot be attacked [acupuncture]; extending [moxibustion] cannot catch up to it; medicinals cannot reach it. It cannot be treated." The Duke said, "You are a good physician." He gave him a generous gift and let him return.
9. 司馬遷《史記》漢.
10. All twenty-five cases are translated in *Pulse Diagnosis in Early Chinese Medicine: The Telling Touch* by Hsu, Elizabeth.

In the post-*Hàn* period, many acupuncture and herbal books began to have case studies sprinkled throughout, for example:

* *Qiān Jīn Fāng* (Formulas Worth a Thousand Pieces of Gold) by Sūn Sīmiǎo (*Táng*),[11]
* *Zhēn Jiǔ Zī Shēng Jīng* (the Classic of Nourishing Life with Acupuncture-Moxibustion) by Wáng Zhízhōng (1220, *Sòng*),[12] and
* the books of Zhū Dānxī and the other masters of the *Jīn-Yuán* period.

These cases were often added as supporting evidence of a treatment or theory's efficacy. Sometimes a strange case was discussed just because it was interesting.

From the Northern *Sòng* dynasty, the middle volume of *Xiǎo Ér Yào Zhèng Zhí Jué* (Proven Formulae of Medicine for Small Children)[13] was entitled *Records of 23 Illness Patterns*. These were twenty-three pediatric cases. It seems to be the first collection like this since the *Shǐ Jì* (Historical Records).

The first book solely dedicated to medical case histories was *Shāng Hán Jiǔ Shí Lùn* (Discussion of Ninety Cold Damage Cases) by Xǔ Shūwēi[14] (c. 1075 - 1156) in the Southern *Sòng* dynasty. This book was not formally published until many centuries later, but handwritten copies circulated freely.

From that time until the mid-*Míng*, few if any new case collections were written, although cases were still included in various medical writings and historical records. Because technology made the printing of books much easier, many *Míng* doctors began publishing their own books, and one popular category at the time was the case study collection.

According to histories, the following books started the *Míng* case study trend:

---

11. 孫思邈《千金方》唐.
12. 王執中《針灸資生經》宋.
13. 錢乙《小兒藥證直訣》宋, published in 1119. This book is usually attributed to Qián Yǐ (c. 1032 - 1113) but the theory, treatments, and cases were actually collected by an admirer named Yán Xiàozhōng 閻孝忠.
14. 許叔微《傷寒九十論》宋.

- *Shí Shān Yī Àn* (Medical Cases of Stone Mountain), by Wāng Jī (c. 1531): This was a collection of his own cases, gathered by his disciples and approved by Wāng.[15]
- *Míng Yī Lèi Àn* (Categorized Cases from Famous Doctors) by Jiāng Guàn (1549).[16] This was an anthology of cases from many doctors.

After this, case study anthologies and collections of an individual doctor's cases became popular even up to the present.

Wāng Jī may receive credit for starting the case study trend in 1531, but *Miscellaneous Records of a Female Doctor* by Tán Yǔnxián was published twenty years earlier in 1511. Could Wāng Jī have seen it? According to Joanna Grant, Wāng (who was from Ānhuī Province) was an avid collector of books. Book sellers brought books from other regions, including from Tán's province Jiāngsū, and Wāng himself travelled a lot. Yes, it is possible that he saw Tán's book, although we will never know.

Tán's Cases

Not counting the prefaces and postscripts, Tán's book is only 36 pages in the old style of printing. It simply contains thirty-one cases, with little discussion of theory. The cases appear in no discernable order, although occasionally two similar cases are adjacent.

The cases usually include the age and marital status of the woman. Unlike some ancient case study books, the name and rank of the patient (or her male relative) were not given.[17] The chief complaint and important signs and symptoms

---

15. 汪機《石山醫案》. See Grant, Joanna, *A Chinese Physician: Wang Ji and the 'Stone Mountain medical case histories'*.
16. 江瓘《名醫類案》.
17. According to Joanna Grant in *A Chinese Physician: Wang Ji and the 'Stone Mountain medical case histories'*, sometimes doctors shared their cases with literati friends when they were well written and contained a good story or used them to solicit patients. If the doctor wanted high-end clientele, he would include as many cases as he could of nobility and high ranking officials. Some ancient cases seem like they are merely an excuse for name-dropping.

are described. Modern case histories usually list every sign and symptom, but in Tán's cases, only the important ones are mentioned. Often Tán closely questioned the patient to try to find the reason for the condition. Many illnesses were attributed to emotions (13 cases) or excessive labor (9 cases). Others involved weather influences such as wind (8 cases). Many of the patients suffered deficiency. Others had eaten things they could not digest or were bothered by other types of food damage (6 cases). Besides this, two were iatrogenic, two had worms or parasites, and the etiology was not mentioned in five.[18] For those thirteen cases due to emotional causes, eight described liver-related emotions (expressed or unexpressed anger), seven had lung-related emotions (sorrow, worry, damage from weeping) and three others mention unnamed emotions or emotions that were hard to categorize.

One might tend to think Tán treated female issues; while she did, she also treated any disorder the female patient might have. There were three cases of lung disorders, three non-reproductive bleeding disorders, nine digestive disorders, six cases of scrofula or other lumps, five cases with rashes or skin disorders, and seven cases with various other conditions (jaundice, insomnia, numbness of the hands, etc.). Thirteen cases involved reproductive or female disorders but out of these, it was the chief complaint for only five; in the rest, female issues were complicating factors (such as a woman with rash due to postpartum deficiency that allowed wind to enter). None of the cases took place during childbirth; Tán was not a midwife.

After the diagnosis was made, the treatment and results were described. Unnecessary information was not included. The terse cases were all about accurate diagnosis and effective treatment.

Only five cases described the pulse image. Most often this was when the pulse was unexpected and therefore changed the diagnosis. Does this mean that Tán did not feel the pulse every time? Yes and no. Based on careful reading, I believe that if the pulse was exactly as would be expected, Tán did not report it. However, another factor is that travel was difficult for women and sometimes Tán

---

18. In Tán's cases, more than one etiology was sometimes cited, so the numbers given add up to more than the number of cases. This is true in the following paragraph as well.

treated a patient based on the intersession of a third party. For example, in Case 31, the patient was comatose and her mother came to Tán. Tán prescribed medicine and the mother took the prescription back home. Wáng Jī also reported cases mediated through a third-party or by correspondence, so this was not unusual at the time. Although not clearly stated, it is possible that other cases of Tán's were also treated in this way. Of course in these circumstances, the pulse could not be read.

The method of diagnosis most often mentioned by Tán was inquiry (14 cases). Inquiry was particularly significant for Tán's patients as communication between a female patient and male doctor had many obstacles. This will be discussed below.

In twelve cases there were statements to the effect that the patient had been treated by other doctors but did not get better. In two cases the doctor actually made the situation worse (one by a botched operation and the other with poorly prescribed herbs). There were also a couple of cases where Tán's original formula did not work well, so she did not spare criticism for herself when warranted.

As for treatment, Tán prescribed herbs for internal use in 29 of the 31 cases. Topical herbs were given four times. Tán performed moxibustion on twelve patients. She used bleeding in one case and gave a medicinal sachet for one patient to wear. Tán never mentioned performing acupuncture.

Twenty-four of Tán's patients were married or widowed (ages 15-69). Five were unmarried (ages 6-19). Two were housemaids (ages 15 and 18), a term that does not reveal their marital status.

Six patients could be characterized as working class or poor; nine had status or wealth. The societal class of the other sixteen was not stated or definitively implied. In the cases where social status was mentioned, it usually related to the medical condition, for example indulgent diet in the wealthy or excessively hard work in the poor.

The patients ranged in age from six to sixty-nine. There were no cases involving infants. The average age was around 30 or 31 years of age. Three were under ten; five were in their teens; seven were in their twenties; eight were in their thirties; four in their forties; three in their fifties; and one in her sixties.

While this book does not bring out any new theories or elaborate treatments, it provides a true picture of how medicine was practiced by educated doctors during the *Míng* dynasty, gives insight into the lives of women, and allows us to recognize one extraordinary woman who became a doctor.

Tán's Sources

Tán listed eight books as sources for her formulas. All were from the *Sòng, Yuán,* or *Míng* dynasties. Two belong to Zhū Dānxī or his disciples, one to a disciple of Lǐ Dōngyuán, and one was a compilation of many formulas but especially those of Liú Wánsù and Lǐ Dōngyuán. This means that half of her sources were related to three of the four great master of the *Jīn-Yuán* dynasties. Twenty-two of approximately thirty-seven formulas she used were in references that were related to Zhū Dānxī.

Of the other four sources Tán used, one was the official *Sòng* dynasty government-published formulary commonly called *Jú Fāng.* Another is one of the first gynecology texts, *Liáng Fāng,* which is from the *Sòng* dynasty. Two are formula books of no particular description.

None of the formulas Tán used were from *Jīn Guì-Shāng Hán* (the *Hàn* dynasty classical medicine of Zhāng Zhòngjǐng), although two were later modifications of classical formulas. The style of using later formulas was probably inherited from her grandparents.

In only one case does Tán mention books that are not formularies (one pulse text and one acu-moxa reference).

For more details on the books mentioned, please see the book appendix.

Tán's Style of Treatment

While of course Tán treated gynecology and postpartum diseases, her cases also included pediatric, external medicine, dermatology, *bì* patterns, and internal patterns related to digestion, insomnia, and cough.

There are three main clinical features:

1. Tán used formulas from later times, not classical *Hàn* formulas. The ingredients were ordinary, not rare or expensive. The formulas were commonly used, straight-forward, and simple. Tán's style was not flashy; her emphasis was on getting the job done. Tán used pills, powders, decoctions, and ointments; she prescribed herbs for internal use and external application.

2. Tán frequently used moxibustion but never mentioned acupuncture. She applied moxibustion in 13 out of 31 cases, using it for internal medicine, gynecology, and pediatrics, as well as for *bì* patterns and scrofula. Tán used bleeding once for a skin condition.

3. Her diagnostic questioning was careful and thorough, and Tán had a good rapport with the patients, so they told her details of their lives that explained their disease etiology. Tán could talk to patients in a way that male doctors could not. Social restrictions and lack of interest severely limited dialogue with male doctors. Patients received empathy and understanding from Tán.

Did Tán Yǔnxián innovate? No, she did not write about anything that could not be found in other books of the time. However the fact that she treated patients and wrote a book about it, her very existence as a woman doctor, broke all the rules.

How Could Women Become Doctors at that Time?

In Tán's case, she was literate and well educated, but as a young child she was directed towards women's work such as embroidery. When her grandfather realized how smart she was, he decided to teach her. She memorized medical texts in the same way all literate doctors in training did at the time. Although not specifically stated, it was likely she was chosen because none of the males in her family wanted to go into medicine and her grandfather had a desire to pass on his knowledge. Even so, Tán was mostly taught by her grandmother, who was also described as being a doctor. One could envision a practice where the wife treated female patients and the husband treated male patients. The prefaces do not describe how Grandmother Rú learned medicine. Did she also come from a medical family or did she learn from her husband?

A Flourishing Yin describes other examples of female doctors, although these women left no writings. It seemed more common for a wife to learn from the husband or a daughter-in-law to learn from the husband's family. In this way, medical secrets would be retained within the family. If parents taught their daughter, any secrets would leave the family when she married out.

In medicine as in many other professions, every member might contribute to the family business. Children could be sent out to gather herbs and the wife might process herbs or make moxa floss. The sons would learn the family business from the father and grandfather. In such an environment, a talented daughter-in-law might learn a lot and eventually began treating as well. But this scenario is more likely for families of hereditary doctors and might not be the case for scholar doctors who would tend toward the standards of the upper classes.

Tán's family was made up of both hereditary doctors and scholars. This had become common during the *Míng* dynasty. It was very hard to pass the imperial exams (which were necessary to become a government official) and a man might fail repeatedly, never passing or only passing when he was older. Because

21

of this, men often had another profession while they were hoping to receive an official post. This may have been the case for Tán's grandfather; the timing of his two professions is unclear, but he was a doctor who also held official ranking in the government. A doctor of the scholarly tradition such as Tán's grandfather may have been more likely to pass along his knowledge to a daughter or grand-daughter than a hereditary doctor; it did not need to remain inside the family since his medicine was based on book knowledge more than secret family formulas that could be lost when the daughter marries out.

The family of Tán's husband did not practice medicine. They were officials and scholars. She never wrote about their reaction to her medical background or whether they supported her in her practice of medicine. At least we know they did not stop her. Tán did not start seeing patients until after her children were older, so she had already completed the main responsibility of a daughter-in-law. Perhaps the family felt Tán's practice of medicine embodied the Confucian virtue of benevolence.[19] Perhaps the wealthier patients gave gifts of value or social alliances. Perhaps the family did not care as long as no trouble came from it. It is also possible that by the time Tán began practicing, she was the oldest female in the household and therefore had a little power within the four walls.

There were undoubtedly many other women doctors in ancient China but they left no record or the record was not preserved. Women doctors are occasionally mentioned in case studies written by men or in other types of literature. One hopes that more of their writings will be found in the future.

Women's Lives during the *Míng* dynasty and how they interacted with male doctors

Life during the *Míng* was quite different from today. Gender roles were strictly defined and enforced. Much of it sounds extraordinarily confining to modern women (and many men as well). However, we cannot judge ancient gender roles by today's standards. Many wealthy women of the time may have enjoyed

---

19. There is a Confucian flavor in Tán's writing and not a hint of Buddhist language.

and preferred the protected life. Their bonding with others in the women's quarters may have been as close as sisters. They did not suffer the stresses and dangers of the outside world. Tán may not have been as unhappy with the restrictions as we would imagine. On the other hand, some of the comments in her preface seem to show a wish for something different; for example she said she made her son publish her book because she could not go out and do it herself.

The gender roles of poorer women were less restricted; for example they could travel outside the home without a male escort. However, their work was often back-breaking and their food inadequate. It is likely that they would have traded some of their freedom for the easier life of the upper classes.

Tán mentioned that anger was a contributing factor to the patient's disease in about a quarter of the cases. She often explained why – the husband wanted a concubine, the husband cheated people, and so forth. In *Míng* dynasty case studies written by males, anger was also frequently mentioned for female patients but no reason was usually given. In reading these cases, one gets the impression that women were simply angry by nature. Tán's cases provide some insight as to the reasons. We can see dissatisfaction brewing under the surface, but we are given the impression that the individual circumstances are at fault in these thirty-one cases, not the role of women in general. Is this the way Tán felt? Or was she reluctant to say more, fearing that her book would not be published or that it would be condemned if she advocated a different role for women? My guess is that the latter is a modern person's view and was not what was in Tán's heart, but we will never know.

At this time, wealthy women could not see a male doctor without having a male relative such as her father, husband, or son present. Modesty was the utmost female virtue. The male doctor questioned the husband, not the woman herself. He might not be allowed to see her face. He needed to ask for permission to feel her pulse. It is unlikely that acupuncture was performed frequently on upper class women as that involved touching. There are records of women refusing medical treatment to preserve their modesty, with death as the outcome. This refusal was not even for a treatment that involved disrobing. The women just did not want any scrutiny of an unrelated male.

Therefore, cases during the *Míng* were not only filtered through the male doctor's understanding, but the reported symptoms were filtered through the husband's words. If the wife was angry because the husband wanted a concubine, would the husband have said so? Even if he did, he and the male doctor would think it perfectly within his rights. This is perhaps why women were perceived as angry by nature in most accounts, not due to circumstances of their lives.

In addition, to sit quietly by while one's own intimate bodily functions are discussed by two males must have been an embarrassing experience. Is it any wonder then that women preferred to see a female healthcare practitioner when they could?

Ancient Female Healthcare Practitioners

During the *Míng*, as well as in other dynasties, there were different types of female health care practitioners. All of the 'job titles' specified that she was a woman. These terms were often used with distain or contempt by male authors and doctors, whether in fiction or medical books. Below is a list of some such terms.

> *lǎo ǎo* 老媼: old woman (but is often used in the context of a healer).
> *ǎo pó* 媼婆 or *wěn pó* 穩婆: midwife, also female examiner of corpses
> *zuò pó* 坐婆: midwife, women who performs an abortion
> *yào pó* 藥婆: herbal granny
> *yī fù* 醫婦: medicine wife (perhaps a doctor's wife but not necessarily)
> *yī pó* 醫婆: medicine granny
> *nǚ wū* 女巫: witch, sorceress, female shaman
> *nǚ yī* 女醫: female doctor

A midwife had lower status because she got her hands dirty, dealing with blood, the placenta, lochia, etc. She used manual skills while the highest level of respect was given to scholar doctors, who besides pulse-taking, only touched a brush and paper to write prescriptions.[20] Words like *granny* or *old woman* might be used for illiterate female practitioners giving home remedies, simple formulas, or single herbs. There was always something scary about a shaman, even if someone decided to employ one. The term that has the highest status here is *nǚ yī* 女醫 female doctor, which is the term Tán Yǔnxián used for herself. Tán was highly literate and had studied the important medical texts. If society had allowed it, she could have debated or discussed cases with male doctors.

Another reason female health care practitioners were not trusted by men is that they had access to the women's inner quarters, an area generally forbidden to males. As described above, for a male doctor to see a female patient (at least within the upper classes), he had to be accompanied by one of the woman's male relatives. The doctor usually questioned the accompanying man. He needed permission to feel her pulse. She might remain hidden behind a bed curtain or veil so even her facial complexion or the form of her body may not be seen.

On the other hand, female practitioners could go into the inner quarters unescorted. They had full access to questioning, pulse, and facial diagnosis. They also could be consulted about abortion, birth control, and so forth. The husband might want control of these, but a female practitioner could circumvent him. These were women who held power that males could not easily restrict.

Tán mentioned inquiry in about half of her cases, and it is obvious that she spent time talking to the patient in many more. One hears stories of doctors who only need to feel the pulse without asking any questions and then they know everything about the patient. However, here inquiry was probably therapeutic as well as diagnostic. Emotions were mentioned for thirteen of the thirty-one cases, with almost as many instances related to sorrow as for anger. These women could pour their hearts out to Tán. Relief came from the medicine, yes, but also from telling their story and receiving the female doctor's empathy.

---

20. A lower status was also given to male doctors who specialized in acupuncture, moxibustion, or treating injuries, sores, and wounds because these involved manual techniques.

In the first postscript, one of Tán's high-ranking male relatives wrote that a female doctor treating female patients "is like the military strategy of 'anything can be overcome when one uses barbarians to attack barbarians.'" The meaning is similar to the English saying of 'fighting fire with fire.' It also implies that, just like one barbarian might understand the ways of another barbarian, a female doctor could also understand female patients better than a male doctor could. But the insult implied is also clear: those with higher status don't need to get their hands dirty by becoming involved with lesser peoples (barbarians and women).

In the same postscript, its author quotes the old saying, "I prefer treating ten men to treating one woman." While we can explain this in terms of the complexities of the female reproductive system, the weight of evidence makes it clear that male doctors found treating female patients rather burdensome, even if they were generally unwilling to empower a class of female doctors to treat them.

With *Míng* dynasty male attitudes like this, is there any doubt that Tán Yŭnxián's patients would find her care a blessing?

Acknowledgments and How This Translation Came About

Some years ago in a workshop at UCLA, I met Charlotte Furth, the author of *A Flourishing Yin: Gender in China's Medical History*.[21] I was quite pleased as I had been fascinated by her book. A few months later, I ran into Charlotte again during a guided hike through Topanga Canyon. She remembered me and we began taking regular hikes through the chaparral together, resting to eat tangerines and discuss Chinese culture and medicine. During that time, she gave me a photocopy of the 1585 edition of *Miscellaneous Records of a Female Doctor*. Charlotte had described this book of case studies, written by a *Ming* dynasty female doctor, in *A Flourishing Yin*. The photocopy remained unexamined until the summer of 2014 when I took it out for no particular reason. I typed up the Chinese for a case study or two and begin translating, just for myself or possibly to use in classes I teach. I was instantly hooked! The patients' stories were engaging and the medicine was interesting. Once I had a rough draft of all the cases, I asked Charlotte if she minded if I publish it, and she generously told me to go ahead. Later she gave me a box of her notes and photos of the one existing ancient copy of Tán's book.

Here is the back-story: During the late 1980s or early 1990s, Dr. Furth was in Beijing, doing research in the rare book library of the Beijing Institute of Traditional Chinese Medicine.[22] This is where she and Dr. Marta Hanson came across *Miscellaneous Records*. At the time, it seems no one else was aware of its existence and no scholars were researching it. Dr. Furth was able to obtain a set of photographs for each page of the book (but it is better not to report how she managed to get these photos). In any case, eventually Furth wrote a number of pages about Tán Yǔnxián in *A Flourishing Yin* and other scholars also begin writing about her later.

---

21. Published in 1999 by University of California Press.
22. Zhōngyī Yánjiùyuàn Běijīng 中醫研究院北京.

I would like to add a few more words about Charlotte Furth. She is a Professor Emerita of Chinese History (University of Southern California) with a number of publications to her credit. One of her specialties has been gender and sexuality in the late imperial era. She has been instrumental in aiding a number of up and coming female scholars of Chinese medicine and her book *A Flourishing Yin* is invariably cited in later works on the topic. She has been mentor and dissertation advisor to many, and often let scholars stay in her spare bedroom for months at a time, making use of her extensive library. Charlotte has generously benefitted me in many ways, one of them being the gift of a carload of books on Chinese medicine when she moved into a different house. While I am not a scholar on the level of the professors and students in graduate school at major universities, Dr. Furth also has been open to interacting with those practitioners of Chinese medicine who have scholarly tendencies, such as myself. I am grateful that she exists in this world and blessed that she has been so supportive of me.

After the seed planted by Charlotte Furth sprouted, I bombarded Yue Lu (translator of other books for The Chinese Medicine Database, such as *the Classic of Supporting Life*) with questions about the text and my translation until she was transformed into an editor and co-translator. The book could never have been completed without her and the uncounted hours she researched questions and corrected my translation.

As always, Jerome Jiang untangled the most difficult phrases and decoded the characters that were impossible for me to read in the old printing.

My publisher, Jonathan Schell was able to track down another rare Chinese edition of *Miscellaneous Records* so that we had a second source to check. Besides this, he spent much time and effort giving a final edit, indexing, laying it out, and designing the cover. As always, Jonathan magically turned a raw manuscript into a beautiful book.

In performing an internet search, I came across David Wayne Landrum's beautiful and sorrowful poem about Tán Yǔnxián. He graciously gave me permission to include it in this volume.

Sarah Zanolini gave suggestions for improvement and caught more than a few typos. Her encouragement and detailed reading vastly benefited the translation and my comments.

Njemile Carol Jones also made useful criticisms for this introduction and has given constant encouragement for this project.

My intent was to make this volume accessible for practitioners of Chinese medicine but to also convey the stories of the women: Tán and her patients. If I did not achieve these goals, the failure is mine alone.

Tán Yǔnxián 1461-1554,

a poem by David W. Landrum[1]

female physician of the Míng dynasty

At 96, I wish I could call forth
the stream of patients, women mostly, I
have healed these years—the tender virgin girls
who came with rashes on their secret parts;
women with periods not right or for whom sex
caused pain; those who could not conceive a child.
Ashamed to open up their treasury
of womanhood to a male physician's touch,
they flocked to me, some with a reddened part
quite easily cured; some with menstrual trials;
others, more seriously, nearly mad
in the aftermath of a difficult birth—
the things the men who practice healing arts
record as "women's complaints." That I was
a wife and mother made me empathize
with them and their distress; and I could cure
the womb, vagina, breasts. My son will cut
the woodblocks for prints of the book I wrote.
The Sayings of a Female Doctor lies
a manuscript. The booksellers will not
publish a text by a woman, even one
who served for years, to whom nobility,
the royal court, the wealthy looked for cures.
Self-published, it might see the light of day.
With no apprenticeship, no study with
a master healer (who must be a man),
I'm scorned. My voice from eighty years spent in
the medicinal arts will cease, will go
unheard, and my advice will quietly die,
unpublished. Slender chance my own copies
will sell. The merchants who run bookshops won't
give up space for my title in their stalls.
These silences—a woman's voice is stilled
not out of death and not from a disease
of body, but of body politic.
I hope healing will come to this soft plague,
this lack of voice, this blockage, this complaint.

1. David W. Landrum is a poet and fiction writer. He teaches literature at Grand Valley State University in Allendale, Michigan. "Tan Yunxian," appeared in *Angle*, Autumn/ Winter, 2014; reprinted in *Cha: An Asian Literary Journal*, June 2014.

Rú Luán's Preface[2]

名醫多稱三吳，女醫近出吾錫山談氏，自奉政君暨配太宜
人，皆善醫。宜人傳於其孫楊孺人。此《女醫雜言》則孺人
之手筆也。

There are many famous doctors in Sān Wú.[3] A female doctor has recently
emerged in my Tán family from Xī Shān.[4] Fèngzhèngjūn[5] joined in marriage
with Tàiyírén[6] and both were good doctors. Tán's grandmother passed the
medicine down to her granddaughter, Lady Yáng.[7] This book, *Nǚ Yī Zá Yán*
(Miscellaneous Records of a Female Doctor), was written by Tán herself.

夫醫在丈夫，稱良甚難。孺人精書，審脈投藥輒應；女婦多
賴保全。又能為書，以圖不朽；活人之心，殆過男子。使由
是而通《內則》諸書，則壺限以裏之事，當更有條格儀節以
傳後也。

Now, it is said to be extremely difficult for a male to be good at practicing medicine. Lady Tán Yǔnxián is proficient in book-learning, examining the pulse, and
getting quick results when prescribing herbs; many girls and women rely on her
to keep themselves healthy. She is capable of writing a book so that [her experi-
ence] won't be lost. Her heart-mind of saving people surpasses that of males.
Our understanding of the duties within the confines of the women's chambers

---

2. Rú Luán (born 1454) was a cousin of Tán Yǔnxián, related through her paternal
grandmother, but the exact relationship is unknown. This preface has no title. It is also
undated but must be from the first printing (1511) as Rú mentioned knowing Tán well.
3. Sān Wú 三吳: a place name. Wú was an ancient kingdom in the region of modern
Jiāngsū. Sān Wú is located in towards the lower reaches of Yangtze (Cháng Jiāng 長江)
River.
4. Xī Shān 錫山: Tin Mountain, a section of Wúxī 無錫 City in Jiāngsū province.
5. Fèngzhèngjūn 奉政君: an honorific title for Tán's grandfather, Tán Fù 談復. From
here on, I will identify him as 'Tán's Grandfather.'
6. Tàiyírén 太宜人: an honorific title for Tán's grandmother. From here on, I will identify her as 'Tán's Grandmother' or 'Grandmother Rú.'
7. Yáng Rúrén 楊孺人: Lady Yáng, meaning Tán Yǔnxián - her husband's family
surname was Yáng. Tán was often referred to as Rúrén (Lady) in the Prefaces and Postscripts. From now on, I will identify her as 'Lady Tán' or 'Tán Yǔnxián.'

comes from various books such as *Nèi Zé* (Inner Regulations)[8] - but additional protocols can [now] be passed on to later generations.[9]

太宜人出吾茹，而孺人與予，為表弟兄，惟深知，故又望之。

Tán's grandmother was from my Rú family and I am a male cousin of Lady Tán; I also respect her because I know her very well.

賜進士第朝列大夫福建布政使司右叅儀前，奉勑兵備漳南僉事，姻生茹鑾書

Awarded Metropolitan Graduate with Honors[10] by imperial order, Grand Master for Court Precedence, Fújiàn Provincial Administration Commission Manager of the Royal Lancers, and Assistant Administrator Commissioner; by imperial appointment Assistant for Military Defense of Zhāngnán, written by Rú Luán who is related [to Tán] by marriage[11]

---

8. *Nèi Zé* 《内則》 (Inner Regulations) is a section of *Lǐ Jì* 《禮記》 (Book of Rites) that discusses the gender role of women.

9. This sentence is a little difficult to understand and translate. It seems to say that the ancient understanding of the duties of women can be updated to include medical practice, with Tán as a model for this new duty.

10. In this translation, job titles are usually rendered according to *A Dictionary of Official Job Titles in Imperial China* by Charles O. Hucker, Stanford University Press, 1985.

11. In this case, 'related by marriage' probably means that they have different family names. In other words, they are related through a female line. As cousins, they would be related by blood.

《女醫雜言》序

Preface to Miscellaneous Records of a Female Doctor

妾談，世以儒鳴於錫，自曾大父贈文林郎、南京湖廣道監察御史府君，贅同里世醫黃遇仙所。大父封奉政大夫、南京刑部郎中府君，遂兼以醫鳴；既而伯戶部主事府君、承事府君；父萊州郡守、進階亞中大夫府君，後先以甲科縣，醫用弗傳。亞中府君先在刑曹，嘗迎奉政府君暨大母太宜人茹就養。

I, Tán, [come from] generations of well-known scholars in Xī [Shān], from my late great grandfather who was awarded Gentleman-Scholar[12] and Investigating Censor[13] of the Nánjīng Hú-Guǎng[14] District; he married into the family of Huáng Yùxiān[15] who was from a long line of doctors from Tónglǐ.[16] My late grandfather was conferred Grand Master for Governance[17] and was an official in the Nánjīng Ministry of Punishments; at the same time, my grandfather achieved medical fame. My father's older brother became a Secretary and a Manager in the Ministry of Revenue.[18] My late father[19] was the Láizhōu Prefect

12. *Wén lín láng* 文林郎 (Gentleman-Scholar): A prestige title for civil officials of the rank of 7a. This sentence seems to refer to Tán Yǔnxián's paternal grandfather's father, named Tán Shào 談紹.
13. *Jiān chá yù shǐ* 監察御史 (Investigating Censor): the most concentrated, broad-ranging investigative and impeaching officials, members of the Censorate.
14. Hú Guǎng 湖廣: A region including parts of Húnán, Húběi, Guǎngdōng, and Guǎngxī.
15. Huáng Yùxiān 黃遇仙: He was apparently a famous doctor who lived in the area. The exact relationship to Tán's great grandfather is unknown.
16. Tónglǐ 同里: A place near Sūzhōu 蘇州. This could also simply mean from 'the same village' - that Tán's grandfather and Huáng Yùxiān were from the same village.
17. *Fèng zhèng dà fū* 奉政大夫 (Grand Master for Governance): A prestige title for civil officials of a certain rank. This refers to Tán Fù 談復, Tán Yǔnxián's paternal grandfather.
18. The name of Tán's uncle was Tán Jīng 談經 according to research done by Zhèng Jīnshēng 鄭金生.
19. Tán Yǔnxián's father was named Tán Gāng 談綱 according to research done by Zhèng Jīnshēng 鄭金生.

and he entered the rank of Lesser Grand Master of the Palace; in a short time he took first place in the third degree [examination] in the county, but the medicine was not passed on to him. My father first worked in the Ministry of Justice and he received my Grandfather and Grandmother Rú [his parents] to live with him.[20]

妾時垂髫，侍側亞中府君，命歌五七言詩，及誦女教《孝經》等篇以侑觴。奉政喜曰：女甚聰慧，當不以尋常女紅拘，使習吾醫可也。妾時能記憶，不知其言之善也。

When my hair was hanging down in the style worn by children, I waited on my father. He ordered me to sing five- and seven-character poems as well as to read aloud from texts such as those on the education of girls or the *Xiào Jīng* (Classic of Filial Piety) in order to entertain him while he drank. My grandfather happily said, "This girl is very intelligent; we should not restrict her to ordinary needle-work but instead we can let her study my medicine." At that time I was able to memorize but I did not understand the value of the words.

是後讀《難經》、《脈訣》等書，晝夜不輟。暇則請太宜人講解大義，頓覺瞭瞭無窒礙，是已知其言之善而未嘗有所試也。

Later I read books such as the *Nán Jīng* (Classic of Difficulties) and *Mài Jué* (Rhymed Pulse Formulas) day and night without interruption. When there was free time, I asked Grandmother to explain the principles and could immediately perceive their brilliance without any obstruction [to my understanding]. This was when I understood the value of the words, but I had never tested them.

笄而於歸，連得血氣等疾，凡醫來，必先自疹視，以驗其言，藥至亦必手自揀擇，斟酌可用與否。後生三女一子，皆在病中，不以他醫用藥，但請教太宜人手自調劑而已，是已有所試而未知其驗也。

---

20. The main point of this paragraph is that Tán came from an elite family of government officials many of whom also practiced medicine. Since her father and uncle did not follow the family medical tradition, it left an opening that Tán eventually filled.

When I was 15, my hair was put up in hairpins and I married, but I continuously suffered diseases of blood and qì.[21] Whenever the doctor came, I would first diagnose myself in order to test what the doctor said. When the herbs arrived, I would also pick through them myself, deliberating whether or not they could be used.[22] Afterwards I gave birth to three girls and one boy. When [the children] were sick, I did not use other doctors' herbal medicine, rather directly seeking advice from my grandmother on modifying the prescriptions and that was all. This was when I tested the medicine a little, but I did not yet understand just how effective it was.

及太宜人捐養，盡以素所經驗方書並治藥之具，親以授妾
曰：謹識之，吾目瞑矣。妾拜受感泣過哀，因病淹淹七逾
月，母恭人錢，私為妾治後事，而妾不知也。昏迷中夢太宜
人謂妾曰：汝病不死，方在某書幾卷中。依法治之，不日可
愈。汝壽七十有三，行當大吾術以濟人，宜毋患。妾驚覺，
強起檢方調治，遂爾全瘳。是已知其驗矣。

Then, when my grandmother was passing on, she personally gave me all her books with formulas of proven effectiveness and the tools for herbal medicine treatment. She said, "If you diligently memorize this, I can die content." I bowed and accepted them. I was moved to tears and overwhelmed by grief. [After that] I suffered a disease that lingered for more than seven months. Because of this my mother, Respectful Lady[23] Qián, secretly arranged funeral affairs for me, but I did not know about it. In a stupor, I dreamt that my grandmother said to me, "Your disease is not fatal; the formula is in a certain book in such and such a volume. Treat yourself according to this method and you will recover within a few days. You will have a long life of 73 years. Your practice will surpass

---

21. This probably means female disorders. Volume 7 of *Dān Xī Zhì Fǎ Xīn Yào* 《丹溪治法心要》 by Zhū Dānxī 朱丹溪 is reserved for female complaints. One of the sections is entitled *Xuè Qì Wéi Bìng* 血氣為病 (Blood and Qì Becoming Diseased). The main topic of this section is abdominal lumps accompanied by menstrual disorders. Tán favored formulas written by Zhū Dānxī, so here she may have been using his terminology for her own illness.

22. It was common for doctors to write a prescription and give it to the family. The family would send the prescription to a pharmacy to be filled. Tán checked the quality of the herbs and the appropriateness of the formula to decide whether or not it was acceptable.

23. *Gōng rén* 恭人 (Respectful Lady): An honorific title for the wife of a rank 4 official.

my skill that has been used to aid people so they don't suffer." I awoke with
a start and forced myself to get up to examine the formula for restoring my
health; then I completely recovered. This was when I understood how effective
this medicine was.

相知女流眷属，不屑以男治者，絡繹而來，往往獲奇效。倏
忽数稔，今妾年已五十，屈指太宜人所命之期，三去其二
矣。竊歎人生駒過隙耳，餘日知幾何哉。謹以平日見授於太
宜人及所自得者，撰次数條，名曰《女醫雜言》，將以請益
大方家，而妾女流不可以外，乃命子濂抄寫鋟梓以傳，庶臆
見度說，或可為醫家萬一之助云爾。觀者其毋誚讓可也。

Female family acquaintances who do not like having a male treat them came in
a constant stream and they frequently obtained unusually good results. Many
harvests [years] have passed by swiftly and now I am already fifty years old. This
is two-thirds of the lifespan predicted by my Grandmother. I secretly lament
that human life is like a sunbeam passing through a crack [life is brief]; I do not
know how many days I have left. I diligently use ordinary days to refer to the
things Grandmother taught me as well as what I have learned on my own and
have compiled a number of cases. I named it *Miscellaneous Records of a Female
Doctor*. I would like to use it to ask for advice from famous doctors. Because
I am female, I cannot go out in public so I asked my son [Yáng] Lián to copy
it and to have blocks carved for printing so that I can pass it on. Perhaps my
subjective opinions can help another doctor in certain cases. I hope the reader
will not sneer at it.[24]

正德五年歳，在庚午春三月既望歸楊談允賢述

The fifth year of Zhèngdé's reign, in the third month of spring of a gēng wǔ year
(1510) on the 16th day of the lunar month, narrated by Tán Yǔnxián who is
married to Yáng

---

24. All of Tán's writing uses very humble terms. In part, writing in past times required
more humility and polite words than in modern times. It is possible that Tán is express-
ing self-doubt, but because she was pushing aside gender roles, she may have used
modesty as a shield against male criticism.

The Cases

Case 1: Vomiting and Coughing up Blood[25]

一婦人，年三十二歲，其夫為牙行，夫故商人，以財為欺。婦性素躁，因與大鬧，當即吐血二碗，後兼咳嗽。三年不止，服藥無效。

The husband of a 32 year old woman was a middleman who cheated people of their money. The wife's nature had always been quick-tempered. Because she strongly vented her anger [regarding his behavior], she immediately vomited two bowlfuls of blood and then also started coughing. These [episodes of coughing and vomiting] lasted three years without stopping; she took medicine but it was ineffective.

某先用止血涼血，次用理氣煎藥，再用補虛丸藥。

I first used a formula to stop bleeding and cool the blood [Sì Shēng Wán, see below]; next I used a decoction to rectify qì [Bā Wù Tāng]; then I used herbal pills to supplement deficiency [Dà Bǔ Yīn Wán].

四生丸（出《良方》）
Sì Shēng Wán (from Liáng Fāng)
Pill of Four Fresh Ingredients

Remove the fresh hé yè and use: 去生荷葉用

shēng dì huáng	生地黃		
biǎn bǎi yè	匾柏葉		
	add 加		
huáng lián	黃連	2 liǎng	74.6 g
shān zhī rén	山梔仁	2 liǎng	74.6 g
xìng rén	杏仁	2 liǎng	74.6 g
bèi mǔ	貝母	2 liǎng	74.6 g

右為末，煉蜜丸如彈子大；薄荷湯食後嚼化。

25. The cases are not numbered in the original, but I have numbered them and added the chief complaint for convenience.

39

Powder the above and make honey pills the size of slingshot pellets. Take them with a decoction of bò hé after eating and let them dissolve in the mouth.

八物湯 （出 《拔粹方》）
Bā Wù Tāng (from Bá Cuì Fāng)
Decoction of Eight Substances
add 加

shā rén	砂仁	1 qián	3.73 g
chén pí	陳皮	1 qián	3.73 g
xiāng fù	香附	1 qián	3.73 g
bèi mǔ	貝母	1 qián	3.73 g

右每服水二鍾，薑三片，食遠服 。

[Boil] each dose of the above in two cups of water* with three slices of ginger. Take it between meals.

* This is not a modern measuring cup; it is probably a teacup. It would be a type of cup found in any kitchen.

Dà Bǔ Yīn Wán (Pill to Greatly Supplement Yīn) (from *Dān Xī Fāng*). She took these formulas and completely recovered.

Notes on Case 1

General Background: Most of Tán's cases begin with an age and a description of the patient as a woman (*fù* 婦) or a girl (*nǚ* 女). The reader should understand that *fù* 婦 doesn't simply mean *woman*; Tán consistently used it to indicate a married woman. When she identified the patient as a *nǚ* 女 girl, it not only implied a younger age but also unmarried status. The distinction has some importance as married women suffer problems related to pregnancy, infertility, and childbirth. We can also use this to understand circumstances that were not explicitly described. For example, Case 5 is "a 19 year old girl" who suffers from scrofula. At the time this was written, it would be normal for her to be married by that age. Her disease is serious enough that it has prevented marriage. On the other hand, Case 15 is a 15 year old 'woman' who had already given birth.

Disease Mechanism: In Case 1, the wife tended to be irritable and she blew up when she heard her husband had cheated people. Anger is very hot and sends qì upward. The heat made blood move recklessly and the rising qì carried blood up, resulting in vomiting and coughing blood.

Treatment: Tán followed the adage: In acute disorders, treat the branch; in chronic disorders, treat the root. While the condition had a three-year history, bleeding is usually considered to be acute or urgent. Therefore, the function of the first herbal formula was to cool the blood and stop bleeding; Tán prescribed a modified *Sì Shēng Wán*. The section on vomiting blood in Volume 5 of *Dān Xī Zhì Fǎ Xīn Yào* says, "*Sì Shēng Wán* from *Dà Quán Liáng Fāng* is quite wonderful [for this]."[26] Zhū Dānxī seems to have been Tán's favorite medical source so his endorsement of this formula would have encouraged her to use it.

Here is the original formula:

四生丸
Sì Shēng Wán (from *Liáng Fāng*)
Pill of Four Fresh Ingredients

fresh hé yè	生荷葉	Use equal portions of each. Mash the herbs and make pills the size of qiàn shí 芡實 (1.0-1.6 cm). Each time boil one pill in water. Remove the dregs and drink while warm.
fresh ài yè	生艾葉	
fresh bǎi yè	生柏葉	
shēng dì huáng	生地黃	
		This formula cools the blood and stops bleeding from the upper *jiāo*. It is used for coughing, spitting, or vomiting blood, as well as for nosebleeds.

Tán modified it to cool the lungs and descend qì. Here is the modified formula:

---

26. 「《大全良方》四生丸甚妙 。」朱丹溪《丹溪治法心要》.

Modified Sì Shēng Wán (for Case 1)
Pill of Four Fresh Ingredients

fresh ài yè	生艾葉	It was to be taken after eating with a decoc-
fresh biǎn bǎi yè	生匾柏葉	tion of *bò hé* and dissolved in the mouth.
shēng dì huáng	生地黃	
huáng lián	黃連	
shān zhī rén	山梔仁	
xìng rén	杏仁	
bèi mǔ	貝母	

Once the bleeding was under control, Tán moved on to rectifying qì. She prescribed *Bā Wù Tāng* (Decoction of Eight Substances) from a book called *Bá Cuì Fāng*. This book exists today but is not available in a modern printing or on the internet. In Case 17, Tán prescribed a formula with the same name but stated that it was from *Dān Xī Fāng* (Formulas of Zhū Dānxī). This raises some questions: Are these two different formulas? Is one of them erroneously attributed?

Until new information comes to light, we will assume that it is the same formula, and that it is *Bā Wù Tāng* from Volume 3 of *Dān Xī Xīn Fǎ*. *Bā Wù Tāng* is simply *Sì Jūn Zǐ Tāng* combined with *Sì Wù Tāng*. Today this formula is more often called *Bā Zhēn Tāng* (Decoction of Eight Precious Ingredients).

The section on coughing up blood in Volume 2 of *Dān Xī Xīn Fǎ* says, "When coughing is extreme, add *xìng rén*, removing the skin and tip [referring to a previously mentioned formula that Tán did not use], and afterwards use *Bā Wù Tāng*, modifying it to regulate and rectify."[27] Note that Tán did add *xìng rén* to her earlier formula, even if it was a different formula from Zhū Dānxī's recommendation.

While the main function of *Bā Wù Tāng* is supplementation, it also regulates qì and blood. After three years of coughing and vomiting blood, the patient surely would have some deficiency as well as counterflow of qì. Tán

27. 咳甚者，加杏仁去皮尖，後以八物湯加減調理 。朱丹溪《丹溪心法》

42

modified *Bā Wù Tāng* with herbs to regulate and rectify qì and cool the lungs.

八物湯
Bā Wù Tāng[28]
Decoction of Eight Substances

四君子湯
Sì Jūn Zǐ Tāng
Decoction of Four Gentlemen

rén shēn	人參	remove the stem
bái zhú	白朮	
fú líng	茯苓	remove the peel
gān cǎo	甘草	honey-fried

四物湯
Sì Wù Tāng
Decoction of Four Substances

dāng guī	當歸	remove the stem, soak in liquor, and stir-fry
chuān xiōng	川芎	
bái sháo yào	白芍藥	
shú gān dì huáng	熟乾地黃	sprinkled with liquor and steamed

Tán's additions

shā rén	砂仁	
chén pí	陳皮	
xiāng fù	香附	
bèi mǔ	貝母	

Boil the ingredients in water with ginger and take it warm.

In her book, Tán never directly mentioned *Sì Jūn Zǐ Tāng* (Four Gentlemen Decoction) by name but the ingredients are included in a number of formulas she used, including this one.

---

28. *Bā Wù Tāng* is more commonly known today as *Bā Zhēn Tāng* 八珍湯 (Decoction of Eight Precious Ingredients).

Finally, once the more acute aspects were under control, Tán treated the root. She used *Dà Bǔ Yīn Wán*, which descends yīn fire and supplements kidney-water. This formula is originally from *Dān Xī Xīn Fǎ*.

大補陰丸
Dà Bǔ Yīn Wán (from Volume 3 *Dān Xī Xīn Fǎ*)
Pill to Greatly Supplement Yīn

shú dì huáng	熟地黃	steamed in liquor	6 liǎng	223.8 g
guī bǎn	龜板	deep fried	6 liǎng	223.8 g
huáng bǎi	黃柏	dry-fried until brown	4 liǎng	149.2 g
zhī mǔ	知母	soaked in liquor and stir-fried	4 liǎng	149.2 g

Grind the above into a fine powder. Steam the powder with pork spinal marrow; make into honey pills. Each dose is 70 pills swallowed with boiled salt water on an empty stomach.
Nourishes yīn and downbears fire.

Dà Bǔ Yīn Wán treated the root of the counterflow qì and the vomiting of blood. The heat of yīn deficiency also caused the patient to be irritable (although the husband did deserve a tongue-lashing). *Dà Bǔ Yīn Wán* was also used in Case 3.

General Background: The reader should note a few things about these cases. As with many case studies in old books, Tán did not list every sign or symptom. She only listed the chief complaint and a few of the more significant disease manifestations. The pulse is not listed in most of her cases; it was only mentioned when it was surprising or important for refining the diagnosis. Another reason some cases might not have pulses listed is that a few may have been long distance cousultations, through intermediaries or correspondence when neither woman could travel. Wāng Jī also performed this type of indirect consultation.[29]

At the time this book was written, tongue diagnosis was not used in any significant way. It started gathering favor a couple of hundred years later

---

29. *Shí Shān Yī Àn* 《石山醫案》(Medical Cases of Stone Mountain, *Míng*, c. 1531) is a record of many of Wāng Jī's cases. He described prescribing for patients he has not seen based on their correspondence or after discussion with an intermediary.

and developed along with the warm disease (*wēn bìng* 溫病) school of medicine.

Case 2: Numbness of the Hands

客船上一婦人，年四十歲，患兩手麻木，六年不愈。詢其病原，云無分春秋晝夜，風雨陰晴，日逐把舵。自得疾以來，服［藥］無效。某以風濕症。

A 40 year old woman [who worked] on a passenger boat suffered numbness of both hands that did not recover for six years. I inquired as to the source of the disease. She said that day after day she held the tiller [steering device of the boat], whether it was spring or autumn, day or night, windy or rainy, cloudy or sunny. Ever since she became ill, she took [medicine][30] but it was ineffective. I judged it to be a wind-damp ailment.

治之灸八穴，遂愈。

I treated it with moxibustion on eight points and she then recovered.

Jiān Yú (LI 15)	肩寓	bilateral point
Qū Chí (LI 11)	曲池	bilateral point
Zhī Gōu (SJ 6)	支溝	bilateral point
Liè Quē (LU 7)	列缺	bilateral point

又服除濕蒼朮湯（出《拔粹方》）。

She also took *Chú Shī Cāng Zhú Tāng* (Eliminate Dampness Decoction with *Cāng Zhú*) (from *Bá Cuì Fāng*).

---

30. The word *yào* 藥 herbal-medicine is missing although there is an empty space where it would fit. This same phrase is used many times in the book, so we can assume it is a printing error and that the missing word is *yào* 藥 herbal-medicine.

Notes on Case 2

General Background: Tán used moxibustion in about a third of her cases. She used bleeding therapy in one case and never mentioned acupuncture. In the moxibustion cases, as was customary in ancient books, Tán stated whether each point was treated bilaterally, unilaterally, or consisted of a single point (for points on the midline). In ancient books, both sides of a bilateral point were counted as two points. Here, four bilateral points were named. Multiplied by two (since both sides were used), there are eight points. In enumerating points, those on the midline or points used unilaterally count as one point.

Treatment: This woman had a pattern of wind-damp *bì*-obstruction due to years of exposure to all types of weather. Moxibustion excels at warming the channels and drying dampness. Because it moves qì and blood, moxibustion can also stop pain ('when there is pain, there is no free movement; when there is free movement, there is no pain'). The same can probably be said for numbness. Rather than simply apply moxibustion on the affected site, Tán selected points of the yángmíng channels (which are especially good at moving qì and blood) as well as points that expel exterior evils.

In addition, Tán prescribed a formula she called *Chú Shī Cāng Zhú Tāng* (Eliminate Dampness Decoction with *Cāng Zhú*) from *Bá Cuì Fāng* (a book that is not generally available today). No formula with this exact name has been found. It could be that the name should be written *Cāng Zhú Chú Shī Tāng* 蒼朮除濕湯 as this is the more common word order;[31] there are at least two formulas by this name. One treats leg qì and the other treats headaches, so perhaps neither is the formula Tán used. Of the two, *Chú Shī Cāng Zhú Tāng* from Volume 1 of *Zhèng Yīn Mài Zhì*[32] is the closest match:

---

31. Formula names often start with the chief herb, then go to the main function, and finally the format (decoction, pill, powder etc.). The first edition of *Miscellaneous Records of a Female Doctor* was hand copied by Tán's son, and the second edition was copied by Tán's grand-nephew. Neither were doctors, so it would be easy for one of them to invert the word order in the name of an unfamiliar formula.
32. *Zhèng Yīn Mài Zhì* 《症因脈治》 (Disease Cause, Pulse, and Treatment) was written in the *Míng* dynasty by Qín Jǐngmíng. It was edited and amended later, in the *Qīng* dynasty by Qín Huángshì 秦皇士.

蒼朮除濕湯
Cāng Zhú Chú Shī Tāng (from **Volume 1** of *Zhèng Yīn Mài Zhì*)
Cāng Zhú Decoction to Eliminate Dampness

cāng zhú	蒼朮	No dosage was given. This formula is listed under headaches due to external contraction.
bái zhú	白朮	
nóng pǔ	濃樸	The source says to add *fáng fēng* 防風 for wind; *shēng jiāng* 生薑 for cold; *huáng qín* 黃芩 for summerheat; *chuān xiōng* 川芎 and *bái zhǐ* 白芷 for dampness; or *zhī mǔ* 知母 and *shí gāo* 石膏 for dryness.
bái fú líng	白茯苓	
chén pí	陳皮	
gān cǎo	甘草	
bàn xià qū	半夏曲	

Another possibility is that *Chú Shī Cāng Zhú Tāng* (*Cāng Zhú* Decoction to Eliminate Dampness) refers to a formula named *Cāng Zhú Tāng* (*Cāng Zhú* Decoction). There are a number of formulas by this name and they treat different things - malaria, sudden turmoil (cholera), and pain. Perhaps Tán added 'Eliminate Dampness' to they title to help clarify which *Cāng Zhú Tāng* she meant, although all of them share this function. Here is *Cāng Zhú Tāng* from Volume 3 of *Dān Xī Zhì Fǎ Xīn Yào*.

蒼朮湯
Cāng Zhú Tāng (from **Volume 3** of *Dān Xī Zhì Fǎ Xīn Yào*)
Cāng Zhú Decoction

cāng zhú	蒼朮	Decoct the above. If cold-damp qì settlles into the body, with heaviness, swelling, and pain, and a withered yellow face, add *má huáng* 麻黃.
huáng bǎi	黃柏	
chái hú	柴胡	
fáng fēng	防風	This formula treats pain in the low back and legs due to damp-heat with a pulling sensation and tension of both rib-sides and inability to turn to the sides from sleeping on the damp ground after dew falls.
fù zǐ	附子	
dù zhòng	杜仲	
chuān xiōng	川芎	
ròu guì	肉桂	

It is possible that this formula was modified to treat cold-damp rather than damp-heat and to remove the focus from the lower body.

Case 3: Flooding and Spotting

一婦人，年三十八歲，得患血崩，三月不止，轉成血淋三年，服藥無效。詢其故，云家以燒窯爲業，夫出自運磚瓦，一日運至二更纔止，偶因經事，遂成此症。某謂勞碌太過。

A 38 year old woman suffered flooding [heavy uterine bleeding] that did not stop for three months; it turned into blood *lín*-dribbling that lasted for three years. She took medicine but it was ineffective. I inquired as to the reason. She said that her family runs a kiln as their line of work; whenever her husband went out, she had to carry the bricks and tiles herself. One day she was carrying them and could not finish until the second watch;[33] coincidentally she was menstruating, and that was when this ailment developed. I said that this is taxation from toil.

用補中益氣湯（ 出《 丹溪方 》 ）加

I used *Bǔ Zhōng Yì Qì Tāng* (Decoction to Supplement the Center and Boost Qì) (from *Dān Xī Fāng*), adding

huáng qín	黃芩	1 qián	3.73 g
xiāng fù	香附	1 qián	3.73 g
dà jì	大薊	1.5 qián	5.6 g

後服大補陰丸，即愈。此後，有患如此疾，婦女五六人，服此皆効。

Afterwards she took *Dà Bǔ Yīn Wán* (Pill to Greatly Supplement Yīn) and then recovered. Later, five or six females who suffered this illness took this medicine and all got good results.

---

33. *Ér gèng* 二更 (second watch): The night was divided into five two-hour watches. The second watch was usually considered to be 9 to 11 p.m.

Notes on Case 3

The Disease and General Background: While *lín* 淋 more often refers to urinary difficulty, it is sometimes used to indicate vaginal bleeding. Its original meaning is to dribble or drip. Here blood *lín*-dribbling seems to be used as a synonym for spotting (*lòu* 漏).

Taxation from toil (*láo lù* 勞碌) is mentioned in Cases 3, 6, 16, 19, 24, and 26. All these women suffered from exhaustion due to heavy work. Mathews defines *láo* 勞 as to toil, to suffer, weary, to make to labor. Taxation is a deep fatigue, deficiency, and damage to the body through excessive activity. This can be though work or play, mental or physical activity. Lifestyle, including poor diet and excessive sexual activity contribute to it. Taxation is a weariness than cannot recover in a short period of time by eating well or catching up on sleep. The damage has gone to the core of the person, so recovery needs long-term attention. *Lù* 碌 means toilsome or laborious. Mathews[34] defines *láo lù* 勞碌 as toilsome labor or bodily labor; Wiseman[35] does not gloss this compound term.

Many of the women in Tán's cases had to work to the point of exhaustion. The woman in Case 3 performed heavy physical labor for many hours each day. Today we might call her pattern spleen qì deficiency with the spleen unable to manage the blood. The condition began with flooding, but as her blood became more deficient, it transformed into spotting.

Treatment: Tán used *Bǔ Zhōng Yì Qì Tāng*, which she attributed to Zhū Dānxī. However, this formula was originally written by Lǐ Dōngyuán. Tán probably knew this, but she used the formula from one of Zhū's books. There are minor differences between the two sources, so the following is *Bǔ Zhōng Yì Qì Tāng* from *Dān Xī Xīn Fǎ*. This formula supplements the middle *jiāo* and raises qì, a treatment principle that is suitable for stopping bleeding due to deficiency.

---

34. Mathews, H.R., *Mathew's Chinese-English Dictionary*, Harvard University Press, 1943.
35. Nigel Wiseman's *Chinese-English Dictionary of Chinese Medicine*, CD Version 04, 2014.

補中益氣湯
Bǔ Zhōng Yì Qì Tāng (from Volume 3 of Dān Xī Xīn Fǎ)
Decoction to Supplement the Center and Boost Qì

huáng qí	黃耆		1-1.5 qián	3.73 - 5.6 g
rén shēn	人參	remove the stem	1 qián	3.73 g
gān cǎo	甘草	honey-fried	1 qián	3.73 g
dāng guī shēn	當歸身	washed in liquor, oven dried	0.5 qián	1.87 g
chái hú	柴胡		0.5 qián	1.87 g
chén pí	陳皮		0.5 qián	1.87 g
bái zhú	白朮		0.5 qián	1.87 g
shēng má	升麻		0.5 qián	1.87 g
gé gēn	葛根	use only if patient is thirsty	0.5 qián	1.87 g
		Tán's additions		
huáng qín	黃芩		1 qián	3.73 g
xiāng fù	香附		1 qián	3.73 g
dà jì	大薊		1.5 qián	5.6 g

In the section on flooding and spotting in Volume 5 of *Dān Xī Xīn Fǎ*, Zhū Dānxī wrote that Lǐ Dōngyuán had methods for treating flooding and spotting but that he did not discuss heat as one of its causes. He recommended that for flooding and spotting due to taxation, *huáng qí* and *rén shēn* should be used but for flooding and spotting due to heat, *huáng qín* was the main herb. These three herbs were all in the formula. Tán added herbs to cool and regulate the blood and to stop bleeding. She did not use a specific formula recommended by Zhū Dānxī but followed many of his recommendations in her treatment.

While the main cause of bleeding seems to be spleen deficiency, we can assume that since the patient worked around a kiln, she was also subjected to a lot of heat. This could also contribute to the bleeding. By starting with *Bǔ Zhōng Yì Qì Tāng* and adding cooling herbs to it, the concept seems to be that deficiency was the main problem and heat was secondary.

In addition, the patient was given *Dà Bǔ Yīn Wán* (Pill to Greatly Supplement Yīn), described in the notes for Case 1. It descends yīn fire and supplements kidney-water. This patient's loss of blood, her long toil, the heat of the kiln, and her age all injured kidney yīn.

Yīn fire is also related to unresolved emotions. While the patient's emotions were not mentioned in the case, one can surmise that she may have resented her husband going out and leaving her with the heavy workload. We don't know the reason for his absence, or whether or not it was for long periods of time, but perhaps he left to do things that displeased the wife.

Case 4: Frequent Miscarriage 1

一婦人，年二十六、七有胎即墮，凡墮六胎，雖服藥不得成，某問其故，其婦性沉怒不發言，火內動之故 。

A 26 or 27 year old woman had been pregnant, but had miscarried six times in total. Even though she took medicine, she was unable to succeed. I asked her about the reason; the wife's nature was to have unexpressed deep-seated anger, so the reason was fire stirring inside her.

遂用紫蘇安胎飲（ 出《 丹溪方 》 ）。

I then used *Zǐ Sū Ān Tāi Yǐn* (*Zǐ Sū* Drink to Quiet the Fetus) (from *Dān Xī Fāng*).

後用
Later I used

yúqián bái zhú˙	於潛白朮	soaked in rice water	2 liǎng	74.6 g
shǔ wěi huáng qín	鼠尾黃芩	vinegar-prepared	2 liǎng	74.6 g

* Yúqián 於潛 is the name of a place near Hángzhōu, in Zhèjiāng province, so this is *bái zhú* from Yúqián.

右為細末，每日空心，紫蘇湯調，下二錢。始得胎安，遂生
一女。

Make the above into a fine powder. Each day swallow two *qián* mixed with a decoction of *zǐ sū* on an empty stomach. The fetus calmed down and she then gave birth to a girl.

Notes on Case 4

Disease Mechanism: In this case, constrained anger led to internal fire. In the past, this had stirred up the fetus and caused six miscarriages. In the section on pregnancy in Volume 7 of *Dān Xī Zhì Fǎ Xīn Yào*, Zhū Dānxī wrote: "Many miscarriages are from [both] internal heat and deficiency in theory. Every day the woman becomes hotter and more deficient. We should determine which is milder and which is more serious. Now it seems that up until the third month of pregnancy, the upper [body] belongs to minister fire [flaring up from below] and as a result it is easy to miscarry."[36] The patient was pregnant again and her anger risked the stirring of minister fire.

Treatment: Tán prescribed *Zǐ Sū Ān Tāi Yǐn*, attributed to *Dān Xī Fāng*. In Volume 7 of *Dān Xī Zhì Fǎ Xīn Yào*, there is a formula called *Zǐ Sū Yǐn* (*Zǐ Sū* Drink). This is probably the same formula as *Zǐ Sū Ān Tāi Yǐn* since it is in the section on quieting the fetus (*ān tāi*):

紫蘇飲
Zǐ Sū Yǐn (from Volume 3 of *Dān Xī Zhì Fǎ Xīn Yào*)
Zǐ Sū Drink [to Quiet the Fetus]

zǐ sū yè	紫蘇連莖	with the connected stems	1 liǎng	37.3 g
dāng guī	當歸		7 qián	26.11 g
rén shēn	人參		0.5 liǎng	18.65 g
chuān xiōng	川芎		0.5 liǎng	18.65 g

---

36. 墮於內熱而虛者，於理為多，日熱日虛，當分輕重，蓋孕至三月，上屬相火，所以易墮。《丹溪治法心要》

bái sháo yào	白芍藥	0.5 liǎng	18.65 g
chén pí	陳皮	0.5 liǎng	18.65 g
gān cǎo	甘草	3 qián	11.2 g
dà fù pí	大腹皮	0.5 liǎng	18.65 g
jiāng	薑		4 slices
cōng	蔥		a length of 7 cùn

Decoct and take on an empty stomach.

There is a second unnamed formula here. Perhaps we can call it *Bái Huáng Ān Tāi Sǎn* 白黃安胎散 (White and Yellow Powder to Quiet the Fetus). Tán also prescribed it in Case 27. This formula consists of powdered *bái zhú* and *huáng qín* taken with a decoction of *zǐ sū yè*. All three of these herbs have the function of quieting the fetus. *Zǐ sū yè* is also used in treating morning sickness. *Bái zhú* and *huáng qín* are a specific combination for restless fetus due to heat and are the basis of a number of Zhū Dānxī's formulas for this condition. In fact, in Volume 7 of *Dān Xī Zhì Fǎ Xīn Yào*, Zhū wrote, "To quiet the fetus before giving birth, *bái zhú* and *huáng qín* are wonderful medicine."[37]

Zhū also wrote in Volume 7, "*Huáng qín* quiets the fetus as it is an herb of both the upper and middle *jiāo* that is able to descend fire and move it downward."[38] And again: "*Huáng qín* is a saintly medicine to quiet the fetus. The common people do not know, taking it as too cold and not daring to use it. They say [only] warm herbs can nourish the fetus; they hardly realize that one should clear heat before giving birth. When heat is cleared, blood follows the channels and does not move recklessly, so the blood is able to nourish the fetus."[39]

---

37. 產前安胎，白朮、黃芩、妙藥也。《丹溪治法心要》
38. 黃芩安胎，乃上、中二焦藥，能降火下行也。《丹溪治法心要》
39. 黃芩乃安胎之聖藥也，俗人不知以為寒，而不敢用，謂溫藥可養胎，殊不知以為產前當清熱，清熱則血循經不妄行，故能養胎。《丹溪治法心要》

Case 5: Scrofula 1

一女子，年一十九歲，患兩頸瘰癧。灸八穴，遂發膿潰，其
根如燈心之狀，其瘡即愈。

A 19 year old girl suffered scrofula sores on both sides of her neck. I applied
moxibustion to eight points and then the sores suppurated. Their roots were in
the shape of a lamp wick. The sores then recovered.

Yī Fēng (SJ 17)	醫風	bilateral point
Jiān Jǐng (GB 21)	肩井	bilateral point
Tiān Jǐng (SJ 10)	天井	bilateral point
Zhǒu Jiān (non-channel)	肘尖	bilateral point

Notes on Case 5

The Disease and General Background: Scrofula (*lì* 癧) or scrofula
sores (*lì chuāng* 瘰瘡) were the diagnosis in Cases 5, 7, and 16. Besides
this, the patient in Case 8 had phlegm nodes in her neck, which belong in
the same category. Scrofula in the modern Western medical sense is tuberculosis or related mycobacterial infections[40] that have progressed from
the lungs into the cervical lymph nodes. Today this is more properly called
mycobacterial cervical lymphadenitis. Manifestations include painless
lumps in the neck that do not decrease in size and usually grow over time.
The lumps themselves are not hot or discolored. When scrofula is caused
by tuberculosis (about 95% of cases in adults), there are usually also fever,
chills, fatigue, and weight loss. As the lumps grow, they may rupture and
form an open wound or fistula; the term *scrofula sores* refers to this. Today
in the West, this is rarely seen as tuberculosis, and is vigorously treated with
antibiotics.

---

40. Tuberculosis is a type of mycobacteria. Other non-tuberculous mycobacteria can
also cause scrofula.

During the *Míng* dynasty, anything with similar appearance and symptoms would be called *lì*-scrofula, even if mycobacterial infection was not the cause. They obviously did not have x-rays, medical labs, or biopsies to confirm the presences of mycobacteria. Besides mycobacterial cervical lymphadenitis, another condition that may have been called scrofula by the ancients would be cancer that has metastasized to the lymph nodes. Today, the lymphadenopathy associated with AIDS would likely fall into this category. Therefore, in these four cases, we cannot be sure that this is mycobacterial cervical lymphadenitis, but we will still use the term scrofula to translate *lì* 癧.

According to Chinese medicine, scrofula is a type of phlegm node. In the section on phlegm in Volume 2 of *Dān Xī Zhì Fǎ Xīn Yào*, it says, "Whenever nodules (*jié hé*)[41] on the human body are not red, not painful, and do not form pus, they are all phlegm streaming [into the channels]."[42]

In Chinese medicine, the main sign of scrofula is phlegm nodes in the neck, armpits, or groin. It is usually associated with lung and kidney yīn deficiency. The heat from yīn deficiency cooks the fluids, turning them into phlegm. The phlegm nodes are not warm (although the patient is warm overall) and are painless. The nodes are hard and immobile. When the nodes rupture, they produce thin pus or occasionally a thicker discharge. The sores heal eventually, although some may form chronic fistulas. In this case, the scrofula lump ulcerated making a fistula which was long and thin like the wick of an oil lamp.

In Case 5, no other symptoms are given, so we cannot speculate whether this scrofula is a mycobacterial infection or some other condition manifesting in lumps on the neck.

The Treatment: Tán used moxibustion as part or all of the treatment in the four cases related to scrofula; in two of these cases, no additional herbal medicine was given. Moxibustion was usually a part of the treatment for scrofula in ancient times. In the section on scrofula in Volume 6 of *Dān*

---

41. *Jié hé* 結核 (nodules): This term usually refers to the tubercles of tuberculosis.
42. 凡人身結核，不紅 、不痛 、不作膿，皆痰注也 。《 丹溪治法心要 》

Xī Zhì Fǎ Xīn Yào, it says, "Externally, applying mugwort moxibustion also gradually obtains results."[43]

The points Tán selected for moxibustion in these four cases are listed in the following table:

Case	Yī Fēng SJ 17	Jiān Jǐng GB 21	Tiān Jǐng SJ 10	Zhǒu Jiān non-channel	Shǒu Sān Lǐ LI 10	Nèi Guān PC 6	Jiān Shǐ PC 5	Jué Gǔ GB 39
5	√	√	√	√				
7	√	√	√		√	√	√	
8	left	left						
16	√	√	√	√	√	√	√	√

Zhǒu Jiān 肘尖 means *tip of the elbow*, and that is exactly where it is located. It treats scrofula and is a moxibustion-only point. Tán prescribed it twice in these case studies: here and in Case 16.

We can see that certain points tend to be used to treat scrofula, but also the treatment varied depending on the patient. Note the prominence of points on the shàoyáng and juéyīn channels. For the details, see each of these cases.

Many old books recommend indirect moxibustion on garlic on top of the scrofula sores or lumps. Tán did not mention the use of isolating substances, so perhaps she only used direct moxibustion. On the other hand, Tán may not have recorded the specific moxibustion techniques she used. Tán also used moxibustion on patients with digestive disorders. Did she burn the cones on ginger slices or use direct moxibustion? We do not know. It is unlikely that she used a moxa stick as these were not common in the *Míng* dynasty.

---

43. 外施艾灸，亦漸取效 。《 丹溪治法心要 》

Case 6: Fire-Cinnabar Rash

一婦人，年四十三歳，其夫因無子，取一妾，帶領出外。婦
憂忿成疾，兩腿火丹大發；又加熱甚，其脈大而極數。醫者
多以憂愁鬱結，治之皆不獲効。

Because a 43 year old woman was childless, her husband brought home a
concubine. He took the concubine out [so people saw, leaving the wife alone
and humiliated]. The wife's sorrow and anger developed into illness with a
great eruption of fire-cinnabar on both legs. She was also very hot. Her pulse
was large and extremely rapid. Other doctors had often treated this as binding
constraint from sorrow and worry, but they never could get results.

某詢其火丹之故，云自為室女時，得此症每遇勞碌、憂忿，
必發不久而退，惟今三月不痊。

I inquired about the reason for the fire-cinnabar; she said that since the time
before she was married, she came down with this ailment every time she was
taxed from toil or when she experienced sorrow and anger. It would erupt and
then fade before long, but now it had been three months without recovery.

某意謂濕毒，治之先用防己飲一帖（出《丹溪方》），其熱
速退。又服一帖，火丹亦退太半，又於火丹紅點處，刺出惡
血。又服前藥二帖，火丹全退。

My opinion was that this was damp toxins; I first treated it using one packet[44] of
Fáng Jǐ Yǐn (*Fáng Jǐ* Drink) (from *Dān Xī Fāng*) and the heat quickly faded. She
then took another packet and the fire-cinnabar again faded by more than half;
I also pricked the red spots from the fire-cinnabar to let out malign blood. She
then took two more packets of the same herbs and the fire-cinnabar completely
faded.

---

44. Pronounced *tiē* or *tiě* 帖 is sometimes used to count the number of packets of herbs.
The text instead uses *tiē* 貼 throughout the book. I have corrected this in the Chinese.
Bāo 包 is also used for a packet of herbs, but not in this book.

又用四物湯二陳湯（出《局方》）加

In another visit I used *Sì Wù Tāng* (Decoction of Four Ingredients) and *Èr Chén Tāng* (Decoction of Two Aged Ingredients) (from *Jú Fāng*), adding:

shā rén	砂仁	1 qián	3.73 g
rén shēn	人參	2 qián	7.46 g
cāng zhú	蒼朮	2 qián	7.46 g
xiāng fù	香附	1 qián	3.73 g

右水二鍾，薑三片，空心服。

[Decoct] the above in two cups of water with three slices of ginger. Take it on an empty stomach.

調理半月而愈。

She took care of herself for a half a month and then recovered.

Notes on Case 6

The Disease: Fire-cinnabar (*huǒ dān* 火丹) is more often called cinnabar-toxins (*dān dú* 丹毒). It is a skin condition that would commonly be diagnosed as erysipelas in Western medicine. A cinnabar-red color quickly spreads on the skin and there are symptoms of intense heat. This case may not be erysipelas - Tán pricked the 'red spots' but erysipelas usually covers a region and would not be described as 'spots.'

General Background: In ancient China, having a son (a male heir) was of paramount importance. Failure to have a son could result in divorce, or the husband could take another wife or concubine to produce an heir. This would obviously cause emotional distress in the wife - both because of her inability to perform her wifely function of producing an heir and because of the intrusion of a new woman into the house. This type of situation could manifest in physical or emotional symptoms.

This Case: At 43, this woman's prospects for becoming pregnant seemed slim, so the husband took on a concubine who was probably much younger. He paraded her around to show her off, adding to the wife's misery. Her overwhelming emotions transformed into heat inside her body and became a rash. Other doctors had simply treated it as emotional constraint. While this was certainly a contributing factor, it was not the complete diagnosis. Tán realized this in part because the previous treatments did not cure her. Upon careful questioning, Tán found out that the rash was recurrent; it erupted with intense emotions, but also with taxation from toil. Therefore, even though it seemed to be a case of pure excess, there was an aspect of deficiency. Tán contemplated it further and came up with the diagnosis of damp-heat or damp toxins. We can assume that the dampness was diagnosed because the rash erupted on the lower body and because it lingered. The damp may have come from spleen deficiency (the taxation) while the heat came from emotional constraint. Tán must have been correct about the dampness because *Fáng Jǐ Yǐn* (*Fáng Jǐ* Drink) cured her.

Treatment: *Fáng Jǐ Yǐn* comes from Volume 3 of *Dān Xī Xīn Fǎ*. It is found under the category of leg qì, and it treats swollen painful legs and feet due to damp-heat. This is an 'off label' use for treating rashes, yet it worked well. The ingredients are:

防己飲
Fáng Jǐ Yǐn (from *Dān Xī Xīn Fǎ* 《丹溪心法》)
Fáng Jǐ Drink

bái zhú	白朮	
mù tōng	木通	
fáng jǐ	防己	
bīng láng	檳榔	
chuān xiōng	川芎	
gān cǎo shāo	甘草梢	
xī jiǎo*	犀角	
cāng zhú	蒼朮	salt stir-fried
huáng bǎi	黃柏	liquor stir-fried

shēng dì huáng	生地黃	liquor stir-fried
xiāng fù	香附	
dà jì	大薊	

* This is from an endangered species and cannot be used today.

This formula has a number of problems from a modern perspective. First, it includes *xī jiǎo* (rhinoceros horn) which comes from a highly endangered species and is no longer acceptable for use in medicine. Besides this, of the two types of *fang jǐ*: *hàn fang jǐ* 漢防己 (Stephania) is acceptable to use, but *guǎng fang jǐ* 廣防己 (Aristolochia) is not due to its content of aristolochic acid. Fortunately, it is likely that this formula would use *hàn fang jǐ*, as that is better at treating the lower body. *Mù tōng* (Akebia) also contains aristolochic acid, which can lead to renal failure. With short term use at an appropriate dosage, these herbs would not have been seen as toxic in ancient times; today, if for no other reason than the legal climate, we should avoid the use of them.

In addition to *Fáng Jǐ Yǐn*, Tán bled the red spots of the rash to further let heat and toxins out. This is the only time in these cases that Tán mentioned bleeding therapy.

After the rash was gone, Tán used *Sì Wù Tāng* and *Èr Chén Tāng* together, adding herbs to transform dampness, regulate qì, and supplement the spleen. This would help to remove the women's predisposition to erupt in rashes by strengthening the spleen and transforming dampness, as well as by regulating and supplementing blood.

Sì Wù Tāng (used in Cases 1, 6, 12, 18, 21, and 31) was originally from *Tài Píng Huì Mín Hé Jì Jú Fāng*.[45]

---

45. This long title of the book is usually shortened to *Jú Fāng* 《局方》. It was compiled and added to by the *Sòng* Imperial Medical Bureau 宋太醫局編, between 1078 and 1085 (*Sòng* dynasty).

四物湯
Sì Wù Tāng (from *Tài Píng Huì Mín Hé Jì Jú Fāng*)
Decoction of Four Substances

dāng guī	當歸	remove the stem, soak in liquor, and stir-fry	Equal portions of each
chuān xiōng	川芎		
bái sháo yào	白芍藥		
shú gān dì huáng	熟乾地黃	sprinkled with liquor and steamed	

Make the above into a coarse powder. Each dose is three *qián* boiled in 1.5 small-cups of water down to eighty percent. Remove the dregs, and take hot on an empty stomach before meals.

This formula is used with modifications for almost every female disorder. Its function - supplementing and regulating blood - is a strategy that is also often used against rashes. It may also help to calm her emotions.

Èr Chén Tāng (used in Cases 6, 8, 12, 21, 24, and 31) was also originally from *Jú Fāng*. While this formula is frequently used to treat phlegm-rheum, here it was likely employed to strengthen the spleen, regulate qì, and transform dampness.

二陳湯
Èr Chén Tāng (from Jú Fāng)
Decoction of Two Aged Ingredients

bàn xià	半夏	wash with hot water seven times	5 liǎng	186.5 g
jú hóng	橘紅		5 liǎng	186.5 g
bái fú líng	白茯苓		3 liǎng	111.9 g
gān cǎo	甘草	mix-fried with honey	1.5 liǎng	55.95 g

Break the above herbs into small pieces. Each dose is 4 *qián* (14.92 grams), boiled in one small-cup of water with seven slices of fresh ginger and one piece of *wū méi* 烏梅. Boil until sixty percent, remove the dregs, and take hot any time.

Sì Wù Tāng and *Èr Chén Tāng* are the two formulas that Tán used the most often, in six cases each. While these are simple formulas, she always combined them with other formulas or modified them. Perhaps this tells us that Tán frequently saw a need in her patients to transform damp, supplement and regulate qì, and nourish and regulate blood.

In this case, here is the complete formula Tán used:

Case 6
四物湯
Sì Wù Tāng
Decoction of Four Substances

dāng guī	當歸	
chuān xiōng	川芎	
bái sháo yào	白芍藥	
shú dì huáng	熟地黃	

二陳湯
Èr Chén Tāng (from *Jú Fāng*)
Decoction of Two Aged Ingredients

bàn xià	半夏	usually cooked with ginger 薑 and
jú hóng	橘紅	wū méi 烏梅.
bái fú líng	白茯苓	
gān cǎo	甘草	

Tán's additions

shā rén	砂仁	cooked with ginger 薑 and wū
rén shēn	人參	méi 烏梅.
cāng zhú	蒼朮	
xiāng fù	香附	

If we consider *cāng zhú* a substitute for *bái zhú*, then this may be seen as a modified *Bā Wù Tāng* (also known as *Bā Zhěn Tāng*; see Case 1). Since the rash erupted when the patient was taxed from toil, supplementing qì and blood would be appropriate once the acute situation was resolved. However, calling it *Èr Chén Tāng* tells us that Tán thought the dampness was more significant than the qì deficiency.

Case 7: Abdominal Lumps and Scrofula

一富家女，年一十二歲，小腹有塊，生於丹田，醫者誤認肚
癰開刀。七年膿水不乾，至一十八歲；兩頸遶腰，皆生腫
塊。某細詢其原，即纏腰癧也。

A 12 year old girl from a wealthy family had lumps in her lower abdomen,
growing in the *dān tián*.[46] A doctor misdiagnosed it as an abdominal abscess
and had opened it with a knife. For seven years up until [now when she is]
18 years of age, the pus did not dry up. Swollen lumps were growing on both
sides of her neck and winding around her waist.[47] I carefully inquired about the
source; it was waist-entwining scrofula.

遂灸一十二穴。其塊漸消，惧開刀瘡口亦愈。

I then applied moxibustion to twelve points. The lumps gradually dispersed
and the delayed [healing of] the open sore from the operation also recovered.

Yī Fēng (SJ 17)	醫風	bilateral point
Jiān Jǐng (GB 21)	肩井	bilateral point
Shǒu Sān Lǐ (LI 10)	手三里	bilateral point
Nèi Guān (PC 6)	內關	bilateral point
Jiān Shǐ (PC 5)	間使	bilateral point
Tiān Jǐng (SJ 10)	天井	bilateral point

---

46. *Dān tián* 丹田 is the region below the umbilicus. In some discussions, a more
detailed explanation might be needed, but here it only seems to signify the location of
the lump.
47. This sentence is difficult to translate. Perhaps it should read "Swollen lumps were
growing that wound around the waist like two 'necks.'" The waist or abdomen is mentioned two other times in this case, but the neck is not mentioned again. However, the
moxibustion treatment resembles what was done in other cases for scrofula of the neck.

又服散腫潰堅湯（ 出《 試効方 》 ）

She also took *Sàn Zhǒng Kuì Jiān Tāng* (Decoction to Dissipate Swellings and Break Through Hardness)[48] (from *Shì Xiào Fāng*)

		remove 去	
kūn bù	昆布		
sān léng	三稜		
		add 加	
jīn yín téng huā	金銀藤花	3 qián	11.2 g
qīng pí	青皮	1 qián	3.73 g

右水二鍾，薑三片，煎服 。

Decoct the above in two cups of water with three slices of ginger and take it.

Notes on Case 7

The Disease: The details of this case are unclear, but there seem to be two problems. The first is a lump in the lower abdomen that was misdiagnosed as an abscess seven years ago. At that time, the doctor lanced it, but it never recovered and continued to ooze for all this time. Apparently the lump grew and entwined the waist. Besides this, she had scrofula in the neck.

Waist-entwining scrofula (*chán yāo lì* 纏腰癧) does not seem to be a common term. A related term is waist-entwining fire-cinnabar (*chán yāo huǒ dān* 纏腰火丹) (see Case 6 for more on fire-cinnabar). While fire cinnabar usually refers to erysipelas, waist-entwining fire cinnabar is more likely to refer to herpes zoster in modern biomedicine. This gives an image of the form or distribution of the lumps. The girl in this case had some kind of lumps winding around her waist similar to the distribution of

---

48. Tán's text wrote *Sàn Zhǒng Dàn Jiān Tāng* 散腫淡堅湯 but the actual name of the formula is *Sàn Zhǒng Kuì Jiān Tāng* 散腫潰堅湯. It has been corrected here.

herpes zoster. We should keep in mind that scrofula in the modern sense is tuberculosis of the lymph nodes. But during the *Míng* dynasty, anything with a similar appearance and symptoms would be called *lì*-scrofula, even if tuberculosis was not the cause. The Western medical diagnosis in this case remains a mystery.

Treatment: Moxibustion was used for the scrofula-like lumps. For a discussion of scrofula and its treatment with moxibustion, see Case 5, above. The selected points were all on the arms and shoulders and are appropriate for the scrofula of the neck although they seem unrelated to the abdominal and waist issues. Still, Tán reported that the lumps shrank and the open sore closed up.

Besides this, the patient took a modified *Sàn Zhǒng Kuì Jiān Tāng* - from Volume 3 of *Shì Xiào Fāng*.[49] *Sàn Zhǒng Kuì Jiān Tāng* treats scrofula and other hard lumps, including after the sores have broken open and begun to suppurate. In addition to treating the scrofula itself, this formula is reasonable for the lump in the patient's abdomen. The ingredients are:

散腫潰堅湯
Sàn Zhǒng Kuì Jiān Tāng (from *Shì Xiào Fāng*)
Decoction to Dissipate Swellings and Break Through Hardness

chái hú	柴胡		4 qián	14.92 g
shēng má	升麻		3 fēn	1.12 g
cǎo lóng dǎn	草龍膽	prepared with liquor, stir-fried	0.5 liǎng	18.65 g
huáng qín	黃芩	prepare half with liquor; use one half plain	8 qián	29.84 g
zhì gān cǎo	炙甘草		2 qián	7.46 g
jié gěng	桔梗		0.5 liǎng	18.65 g
lián qiáo	連翹		3 qián	11.2 g
guā lóu gēn	瓜蔞根	slice and smash, prepared with liquor	0.5 liǎng	18.65 g
dāng guī wěi	當歸尾		2 qián	7.46 g
bái sháo yào	白芍藥		2 qián	7.46 g

49. The full name of the book is *Dōng Yuán Shì Xiào Fāng* 《東垣試效方》 by Luó Qiānfǔ 羅謙甫 (*Yuán* dynasty), a disciple of Lǐ Dōngyuán 李東垣.

huáng bǎi	黃柏	prepared with liquor	0.5 liǎng	18.65 g
zhī mǔ	知母	first cut, prepared with liquor	0.5 liǎng	18.65 g
gé gēn	葛根		2 qián	7.46 g
huáng lián	黃連		1 qián	3.73 g
jīng sān léng	京三棱	prepared with liquor, lightly stir-fried	3 qián	11.2 g
guǎng róng	廣莪	cut and smashed, prepared with liquor, lightly stir-fried	3 qián	11.2 g
kūn bù	昆布	remove the dirt	0.5 liǎng	18.65 g

Break the above into small bits. Each dose is 6 or 7 *qián* (22.38 - 26.11 grams) in 2.8 cups of water. Let it soak half a day, boil down to 1 cup, remove the dregs and take it.

Tán removed the *kūn bù* and *sān léng*; she added *jīn yín téng huā* (3 *qián* or 11.2 grams) and *qīng pí* (1 *qián* or 3.73 grams). So with the modifications, it looks like this:

散腫潰堅湯
Modified *Sàn Zhǒng Kuì Jiān Tāng*
Decoction to Dissipate Swellings and Break Through Hardness

chái hú	柴胡		4 qián	14.92 g
shēng má	升麻		3 fēn	1.12 g
cǎo lóng dǎn	草龍膽	prepared with liquor, stir-fried	0.5 liǎng	18.65 g
huáng qín	黃芩	prepare half with liquor; use one half plain	8 qián	29.84 g
zhì gān cǎo	炙甘草		2 qián	7.46 g
jié gěng	桔梗		0.5 liǎng	18.65 g
lián qiáo	連翹		3 qián	11.2 g
guā lóu gēn	瓜蔞根	slice and smash, prepared with liquor	0.5 liǎng	18.65 g
dāng guī wěi	當歸尾		2 qián	7.46 g
bái sháo yào	白芍藥		2 qián	7.46 g
huáng bǎi	黃柏	prepared with liquor	0.5 liǎng	18.65 g
zhī mǔ	知母	first cut, prepared with liquor	0.5 liǎng	18.65 g
gé gēn	葛根		2 qián	7.46 g
huáng lián	黃連		1 qián	3.73 g
guǎng róng	廣莪	cut and smashed, prepared with liquor, lightly stir-fried	3 qián	11.2 g

jīn yín téng	金銀藤	remove the dirt	3 qián	11.2 g
huā	花			
qīng pí	青皮		1 qián	3.73 g
				3 slices

Decocted with ginger 薑.

Case 8: Phlegm Nodes

一婦人，年三十二歲，左頸患痰核。與灸二穴。

A 32 year old woman suffered from phlegm nodes on the left side of her neck. I gave her moxibustion on two points.

Yī Fēng (SJ 17)	醫風	one point on the left
Jiān Jǐng (GB 21)	肩井	one point on the left

又服當歸連翹湯（出《袖珍方》）加二陳湯。

She also took *Dāng Guī Lián Qiáo Tāng* (Decoction of *Dāng Guī* and *Lián Qiáo*) (from *Xiù Zhēn Fāng*) adding *Èr Chén Tāng* and

cāng zhú	蒼朮	2 qián	7.46 g
qīng pí	青皮	1 qián	3.73 g

右水二鍾，薑三片。服之十帖，此核遂消。

Decoct the above in two cups of water with three slices of ginger. She took ten packets and the nodes then dispersed.

Notes on Case 8

Treatment: Moxibustion was used for the patient's phlegm nodes (see Case 5 regarding scrofula, above). Phlegm node is usually a synonym for scrofula, especially when it has not ulcerated. Most of Tán's scrofula cases had swollen nodes on both sides and moxibustion was applied bilaterally. This one manifested on the left side only, so moxibustion was given only on the affected side.

Dāng Guī Lián Qiáo Tāng (from *Xiù Zhēn Fāng*) was combined with *Èr Chén Tāng* (see Case 6); *cāng zhú* (two *qián*) and *qīng pí* (one *qián*) were also added.

Here, *Dāng Guī Lián Qiáo Tāng* is attributed to *Xiù Zhēn Fāng* (Pocket-Size Formulary). Unfortunately, no copy of the formula is available from the named source. It seems the formula name should actually be *Dāng Guī Lián Qiáo Sǎn* 當歸連翹散 (not *Tāng* 湯).[50] Looking at other sources for formulas named *Dāng Guī Lián Qiáo Sǎn*, Volume 1 of *Chuāng Yáng Jīng Yàn Quán Shū*[51] seems the closest match to Tán's patient:

50. The full name of the book is *Xiù Zhēn Fāng Dà Quán* (Pocket-Size Formula Collection) 《袖珍方大全》. The author was Lǐ Héng 李恒 et al.. It has four volumes and was published in 1391 (*Míng*). This book is a compilation of useful formulas from other sources. While copies of this book still exist, there seems to be no modern printing, and no electronic copies were found in an internet search. Yue Lu was able to obtain a .pdfed scan of portions of an ancient edition. Unfortunately, the section with this formula was not included in the scan. However, the table of contents lists *Dāng Guī Lián Qiáo Sǎn* 當歸連翹散 (not *Tāng* 湯) in Volume 3 under the heading of abscesses and sores. It may have been called *Tāng* (decoction) here because it was boiled in water. Many *Sǎn* (powder) formlas are decocted after they are powdered, adding to the confusion in names.
51. *Chuāng Yáng Jīng Yàn Quán Shū* 《瘡瘍經驗全書》 is an external medicine (*wài kē*) work of 13 volumes. It was attributed to Dòu Hànqīng 竇漢卿 of the *Sòng* dynasty but it was really written by Dòu Mènglín 竇夢麟 in 1569 (*Míng*). While this book was published later than the time of these cases, it is likely that this or similar formulas were used when Tán was active, less than a century before.

當歸連翹散
Dāng Guī Lián Qiáo Sǎn
(from *Volume 1 of Chuāng Yáng Jīng Yàn Quán Shū*)
Powder of Dāng Guī and Lián Qiáo

dāng guī	當歸	Dosage was not given. Powder the herbs and boil in water with some *dēng xīn* 燈心. Take it orally.
shēng dì huáng	生地黃	
lián qiáo	連翹	This formula treats throat-locking sores that resemble the initial stages of scrofula, with inability to eat or drink because the throat is closed off. The sores gradually swell until they break open and transforms into pus.
qián hú	前胡	
gān cǎo	甘草	
zhǐ qìao	枳殼	
jié gěng	桔梗	
huáng qín	黃芩	
shǔ nián zǐ	鼠粘子	
xuán shēn	玄參	
tiān huā fèn	天花粉	
bái sháo	白芍	

Tán modified the formula. Here is the final form:

Case 8
當歸連翹散
Dāng Guī Lián Qiáo Sǎn
Powder of Dāng Guī and Lián Qiáo

dāng guī	當歸	
shēng dì huáng	生地黃	
lián qiáo	連翹	
qián hú	前胡	
gān cǎo	甘草	also in *Èr Chén Tāng*
zhǐ qìao	枳殼	
jié gěng	桔梗	
huáng qín	黃芩	
shǔ nián zǐ	鼠粘子	
xuán shēn	玄參	

| tiān huā fěn | 天花粉 | |
| bái sháo | 白芍 | |

二陳湯
Èr Chén Tāng
Decoction of Two Aged Ingredients

bàn xià	半夏	wash with hot water seven times
jú hóng	橘紅	
bái fú líng	白茯苓	
gān cǎo	甘草	also in *Dāng Guī Lián Qiáo Sǎn*

Tán's additions

| cāng zhú | 蒼朮 | |
| qīng pí | 青皮 | |

Decocted with ginger 薑.

No other symptoms were given for this case, so it is hard to comment further.

Case 9: Postpartum Sores and *Lài*

一婦人，年二十三歲，患滿身瘡癩，不能舉步痛癢，不可忍。某詢其居處，所居不蔽風日。產後，漸得此瘡疾，一年不愈。某謂產後氣血未和，乘虛被風，搏於皮膚之間，故發此症。

A 23 year old woman suffered sores and *lài* over her entire body with inability to walk and unbearable pain and itching. I inquired as to her dwelling; where she lived did not provide shelter from the wind or sun. After giving birth, she gradually developed this disease of sores and did not recover for a year. I said it was postpartum qì and blood disharmony. This ailment occurred because wind took advantage of her deficiency and swirled between the layers of the skin.

付人參敗毒散（出《局方》）加

I gave her *Rén Shēn Bài Dú Săn* (*Rén Shēn* Powder to Overcome Pathogenic Influences) (from *Jú Fāng*) adding

lián qiáo	連翹	1 qián	3.73 g
jīn yín téng huā	金銀藤花	2 qián	7.46 g
tiān má	天麻	1 qián	3.73 g

右水二鍾，薑三片，煎服。

Decoct the above in two cups of water with three slices of ginger and take it.

又搽藥合掌散（出《摘玄方》）。十日即愈。

She also applied medicine topically: *Hé Zhăng Săn* (Join the Palms Powder) (from *Zhāi Xuán Fāng*). She recovered in ten days.

Notes on Case 9

The Disease: *lài* 癩 can correspond to the Western medical diagnosis of leprosy, but it also includes conditions such as scabies, ringworm, and mange. *Lài* conditions often involve hair loss. In this case, it is not likely to refer to leprosy; itching is not a symptom of leprosy although numbness is.

Wind is often able to enter the body when deficiency leaves hollow areas and crevices between the layers of the skin and flesh. When there is adequate qì and blood, the hollows and crevices are filled and there is no space for the wind to enter.

Treatment: Tăn gave a decoction to expel the evils and strengthen the body and a formula for external application to treat the rash.

Rén Shēn Bài Dú Săn is from *Jú Fāng*. It treats cold damage and seasonal qì and is given to patients with deficiency, including postpartum women.

One of its indications is to treat early stage measles, but other rashes are not mentioned.

人參敗毒散

Rén Shēn Bài Dú Sǎn (from *Jú Fāng* 《局方》)

Rén Shēn Powder to Overcome Pathogenic Influences

chái hú	柴胡	remove the sprouts
gān cǎo	甘草	pound into a pulp
jié gěng	桔梗	
rén shēn	人參	remove the stem
chuān xiōng	川芎	
fú líng	茯苓	remove the peel
zhǐ qiào	枳殼	remove the interior part, stir-fry in wheat bran
qián hú	前胡	remove the sprouts, wash
qiāng huó	羌活	remove the sprouts
dú huó	獨活	remove the sprouts

Make a coarse powder with 30 *liǎng* (1119 grams) of each of the above herbs. Each dose is 2 *qián* (7.46 grams) boiled in a small-cup of water together with a little fresh ginger and *bò hé*. Boil until seventy percent, remove the dregs, and take any time. When there is a lot of coldness, drink it while it is hot; when there is a lot of heat, drink it warm.

Tán added *lián qiáo* (1 *qián* or 3.73 grams), *jīn yín téng huā* (2 *qián* or 7.46 grams), and *tiān má* (1 *qián* or 3.73 grams).

The patient also applied medicine topically: *Hé Zhǎng Sǎn*. Its listed source, *Zhāi Xuán Fāng*, is no longer extant. A number of formulas named *Hé Zhǎng Sǎn* exist, but a probable candidate is from Volume 28 of *Pǔ Jì Fāng* (Formulas for Universal Relief).[52]

---

52. *Pǔ Jì Fāng* 《 普濟方 》 (Formulas for Universal Relief) was sponsored by the *Míng* government and was published in 1406.

合掌散
Hé Zhǎng Sǎn (from *Pǔ Jì Fāng* 《普濟方》 Volume 28)
Join the Palms Powder

qiāng huó	羌活	Powder together equal portions of each of the above herbs.
dú huó	獨活	Mix with the dregs of sesame oil and smear on the palms of the hands. Rub the hands together until it is warm and you
liú huáng	硫黃	can smell it. Then rub it on the sores. It treats scabies (or
qīng fěn	輕粉	scabby sores, *jiè chuāng* 疥瘡).

Qīng fěn (calomelas) is made from mercury, so it is no longer in use today. It was used in the past for scabies and some types of sores.

Case 10: Diarrhea

一富家婦，年三十三歲，患泄瀉，服藥無効。詢其故，飲食
太過，不能尅化。此為脾家久受虛濕所致。用艾火灸，五
穴。其瀉漸止。又服和胃白朮丸（出《摘玄方》）。

A 33 year old woman from a wealthy household suffered diarrhea; she took medicine but without results. I inquired as to the reason; she had overindulged in food and drink and was unable to digest it. This was caused by deficiency of the spleen with dampness that had been present for a long time. I used mugwort fire moxibustion on five points. Her diarrhea gradually ceased. She later took *Hé Wèi Bái Zhú Wán* (*Bái Zhú* Pill to Harmonize the Stomach) (from *Zhāi Xuán Fāng*).

Shàng Wǎn (Rèn 13)	上脘	single point
Zhōng Wǎn (Rèn 12)	中脘	single point
Xià Wǎn (Rèn 10)	下脘	single point
Tiān Shū (ST 25)	天樞	bilateral point

至八月復灸 。

Upon reaching the eighth lunar month [around September in the Western calendar] we again applied moxibustion.

Gāo Huāng (UB 43)	膏肓	bilateral point
Pí Shù (UB 20)	脾腧	bilateral point
Dà Zhuì (Dū 14)	大椎	single point
Sān Lǐ (ST 36)	三里	bilateral point

遂獲全愈 。

Then she was able to recover completely.

Notes on Case 10

Treatment: The first moxibustion formula Tán used is similar to the treatment in other cases in which the patient could not easily take herbs: vomiting, difficulty swallowing, or diarrhea (Cases 10, 11, 13, 21). With diarrhea, the patient could drink the herbs, but they would not remain in the body long enough to be absorbed. In Case 25, Tán also used similar moxibustion points for a lump in the abdomen that had been there a long time. In all these cases, she applied moxibustion on the three wǎn - Shàng Wǎn (Rèn 13), Zhōng Wǎn (Rèn 12), and Xià Wǎn (Rèn 10) - plus one other point which varied from case to case.

Case	Complaint	Shàng Wǎn Rèn 13	Zhōng Wǎn Rèn 12	Xià Wǎn Rèn 10	Other Point
10	diarrhea	√	√	√	Tiān Shū (ST 25)
11	diarrhea	√	√	√	Shí Guān (non-channel)
13	vomiting, emaciation	√	√	√	Shí Guān (non-channel
21	diaphragm qì	√	√	√	Shí Guān (non-channel)

25	abdominal lump	√	√	√	Lóng Xìng (non-channel)

In this case (Case 10), Tán applied moxibustion on these points to stop the diarrhea. After the diarrhea stopped, Tán changed the point formula to supplement the patient's chronic spleen deficiency. At that time, the treatment focused on treating the root. This treatment occurred in the eighth lunar month, which contains the autumn equinox. Perhaps Tán wanted to give the patient a boost before the onset of winter.

This patient also took an herbal formula, *Hé Wèi Bái Zhú Wán* (from the lost book *Zhāi Xuán Fāng*[53]) which is also used in Cases 13 and 22. It probably refers to *Bái Zhú Hé Wèi Wán* (Bái Zhú Pill to Harmonize the Stomach), which was originally from *Nèi Wài Shāng Biàn*.[54] Here is another time the word order in the name of the formula seems to be inverted (see also Case 2).

The name of the formula

Hé Wèi 和胃 ↘	Bái Zhú 白朮	Wán 丸	The name given by Tán
Bái Zhú 白朮 ↗	Hé Wèi 和胃	Wán 丸	The probable name
These two pairs of words are inverted		Pills	

Here is *Bái Zhú Hé Wèi Wán* from *Nèi Wài Shāng Biàn*:

白朮和胃丸
Bái Zhú Hé Wèi Wán (from *Nèi Wài Shāng Biàn* 《內外傷辨》)
Bái Zhú Pill to Harmonize the Stomach

bái zhú	白朮		1.2 liǎng	44.76 g
bàn xià	半夏	washed in hot water seven times	1 liǎng	37.3 g
nóng pǔ	濃樸	prepared with ginger	1 liǎng	37.3 g
chén pí	陳皮	remove the white	8 qián	29.84 g

53. The full title of the book is *Dān Xī Zhāi Xuán Fāng* 《丹溪摘玄方》 (*Yuán* dynasty).

54. *Nèi Wài Shāng Biàn* 《內外傷辨》 was written by Lǐ Dōngyuán 李東垣 (1231).

rén shēn	人參		7 qián	26.11 g
gān cǎo	甘草	honey-fried	3 qián	11.2 g
zhǐ shí	枳實	stir-fried in wheat bran	2.5 qián	9.3 g
bīng láng	檳榔		2.5 qián	9.3 g
mù xiāng	木香		1 qián	3.73 g

Make the above into a fine powder. Soak the powder with fresh ginger juice and steam into cakes to make pills the size of *wú tóng zǐ* 梧桐子 (about 0.6-0.9 centimeters in diameter), each dose is 30 pills swallowed with warm boiled water, between meals.

This formula treats stomach qì deficiency. Taking it often harmonizes the center, rectifies qì, disperses phlegm, removes dampness, harmonizes the spleen and stomach, and allows one to eat and drink.

Case 11: Pediatric Diarrhea

一富家女，年方八歲，患白瀉。醫者誤為疳瀉，一年不愈。細詢其故，此女後母所出。某謂愛過，必為食傷。用火灸五穴。又服保和丸一料（出《摘玄方》）。其瀉即愈。

A girl from a wealthy family had just turned eight years old when she suffered from white diarrhea. A doctor misdiagnosed it as *gān* diarrhea and she had not recovered in a year. I carefully inquired as to the reason; this girl was born to a second wife.[55] I said it was excessive love [meaning the girl was spoiled] that became food damage. I used fire moxibustion on five points. She later took one batch of *Bǎo Hé Wán* (Pill to Preserve Harmony) (from *Zhāi Xuán Fāng*). Her diarrhea then recovered.

Shàng Wǎn (Rèn 13)	上脘	single point*
Zhōng Wǎn (Rèn 12)	中脘	single point
Xià Wǎn (Rèn 10)	下脘	single point
Shí Guān (non-channel)	食關	bilateral point

*The original text says bilateral point 二穴. This has been corrected here.

---

55. *Hòu mǔ* 後母 usually means step-mother, but how can a girl be born to her step-mother? It is more likely that she was born to a lower ranking wife who spoiled her.

Notes on Case 11

The Disease: The girl was doted upon by her mother so her diet was not regulated. This lead to diarrhea which had been misdiagnosed as *gān*.

Gān diarrhea (*gān xiè* 疳瀉): English books usually translate *gān* as *infantile malnutrition*. This condition can include parasites, starvation, or various disorders where nutrients are not being absorbed. Diarrhea is a common symptom of *gān*.

White diarrhea (*bái xiè* 白瀉) is a pediatric disorder. The stool is white and thin, with abdominal distention and pain, and pale lips. It is due to spleen-stomach qì deficiency with dampness. It was first mentioned in *Zhōng Zàng Jīng*.[56]

Tán used moxibustion rather than herbs, which might pass through with the diarrhea. Various books locate the Shí Guān point 1.5 cun lateral to either Zhōng Wǎn (Rèn 12) or Jiàn Lǐ (Rèn 11). It is used to treat digestive disorders such as choking on food, stomach reflux, or non-transformation of food. It was first mentioned in *Yī Jīng Xiǎo Xué* 劉純《 醫經小學 》 by Liú Chún, published in 1388 (*Míng*). Tán prescribed Shí Guān three times in these case studies (Cases 11, 13, and 21). For discussion of the moxibustion treatment, see Case 10.

Waiting until the diarrhea was a little better, Tán switched to herbal medicine and used *Bǎo Hé Wán*. She took it from *Zhāi Xuán Fāng*,[57] but here is the recipe from *Dān Xī Xīn Fǎ*:

---

56. *Zhōng Zàng Jīng* 《 中藏經 》 (Classic of the Central Viscera) was attributed to Huá Tuó. It was surely written later, but the time it was written is unknown.
57. A lost text associated with Zhū Dānxī.

保和丸
Bǎo Hé Wán (from Dān Xī Xīn Fǎ)
Pill to Preserve Harmony

shān zhā	山楂	6 liǎng	223.8 g
shén qū	神麴	2 liǎng	74.6 g
bàn xià	半夏	3 liǎng	111.9 g
fú líng	茯苓	3 liǎng	111.9 g
chén pí	陳皮	1 liǎng	37.3 g
lián qiáo	連翹	1 liǎng	37.3 g
lái fú zǐ	萊菔子	1 liǎng	37.3 g

Powder the above. Make into pills the size of *wú tóng zǐ* 梧桐子 (about 0.6-0.9 centimeters in diameter). Each dose is 70 or 80 pills between meals, taken with hot water. It treats all types of food accumulations.

If spleen qì cannot ascend because food accumulations obstruct the qì mechanism, diarrhea may result. The herbs in this formula regulate the qì mechanism and transform stagnant food. By eliminating dampness of the spleen, *fú líng* also helps eliminate the diarrhea. This formula is gentle enough for use in children and can be given in mild cases. However, in cases where old food has been stuck in the digestive track without moving for a long time, it does not have the power to break through. See also Cases 28 and 29.

Case 12: *Nüè*-Malarial Dysentery during Pregnancy

一婦人，年二十一歲，初受胎，六箇月，患疊日瘧痢，將三月。某詢其故，云偶食雞麵，彼翁姑嗔責，遂得此症。先付安胎和氣之劑，服之無効。後服二陳湯，加：

It was the sixth month of a 21 year old woman's first pregnancy; for almost three months she had suffered many days of *nüè*-malarial dysentery. I inquired as to the reason; she said she happened to eat chicken and noodles and her parents-in-law scolded her. That was when she got this ailment. I first gave her a prescription to calm the fetus and harmonize qì; she took it but without results. Next she took *Èr Chén Tāng*, adding:

xiāng fù	香附	1 qián	3.73 g
shén qū	神麴	1 qián	3.73 g
shā rén	砂仁	1 qián	3.73 g
mù xiāng	木香	3 fēn	1.12 g
cāng zhú	蒼朮	1 qián	3.73 g
hòu pǔ	厚朴	1 qián	3.73 g
chái hú	柴胡	1 qián	3.73 g

服之稍可，得九箇月產，下死胎 。

She took it and was slightly better. She was able to give birth after nine months, but the baby was stillborn.

其婦將危，瘧痢復作急 。與四物湯，加：

The woman was near death as the *nüè*-malarial dysentery had relapsed and became acute. I gave her *Sì Wù Tāng*, adding:

xuán hú suǒ	玄胡索		1 qián	3.73 g
bái zhú	白朮		2 qián	7.46 g
chén pí	陳皮		2 qián	7.46 g
shén qū	神麴	dry-fried	1 qián	3.73 g
hēi gān jiāng	黑乾薑		1 qián	3.73 g
xiāng fù	香附		2 qián	7.46 g
shā rén	砂仁		1 qián	3.73 g
cāng zhú	蒼朮		1 qián	3.73 g
hòu pǔ	厚朴		2 qián	7.46 g
cǎo guǒ	草菓		1 qián	3.73 g

服之，瘧痢稍緩，米飲加進後 。

She took it and recovered somewhat from the *nüè*-malarial dysentery, and after swallowed some rice drink.[58]

又付藥六帖：

In another visit I gave her six packets [more of the above] herbs:

	removing 去		
xuán hú suǒ	玄胡索		
hēi gān jiāng	黑乾薑		
	adding 加		
rén shēn	人參	1 qián	3.73 g
mù xiāng	木香	3 fēn	1.12 g
fú líng	茯苓	2 qián	7.46 g
chén pí	陳皮	1 qián	3.73 g*

* This is a bit unclear. *Chén pí* is already listed above so there is no need to add it, unless this means increasing the dosage by 1 *qián* (making a total of 3 *qián* or 11.19 grams) or decreasing the dosage to 1 *qián* (3.73 grams).

又服蒙薑黃連丸（ 出《 摘玄方 》 ）。其病即愈 。

In another visit she took *Méng Jiāng Huáng Lián Wán* (from *Zhāi Xuán Fāng*) and her disease recovered.

Notes on Case 12

The Disease: We can assume that the patient also suffered other symptoms of malaria, such as recurrent periods of fever and chills, headaches, muscle aches, fatigue, nausea, and vomiting. Today, it seems hard to accept that a scolding could cause this. We should remember that the term *nüè*-malaria may have had a wider scope than only the mosquito-borne illness,

---

58. *Mǐ yǐn* 米飲 (rice drink): This is thin rice soup.

although it is possible that this case was due to the biomedicine category of *Plasmodium* infection. In modern medicine, it is acknowledged that malaria can cause low birth weight babies, fetal death, maternal anemia, and other problems. These effects are more severe in first pregnancies. Malaria is still a problem today in Jiāngsū Provence, the region where Tán lived.

Diarrhea or dysentery can be one of the symptoms of *nüè*-malaria. In some ancient books,[59] *nüè*-malarial dysentery was sometimes associated with pregnancy and the postpartum period.

Treatment: Tán's first prescription did not get any results. Next *Èr Chén Tāng* was modified with herbs to regulate qì, dry dampness, and harmonize the shàoyáng. However, this formula had only minimum success as the baby was stillborn and the patient remained ill:

Case 12a

二陳湯

Èr Chén Tāng (from *Jú Fāng*)

Decoction of Two Aged Ingredients

bàn xià	半夏	wash with hot water seven times	5 liǎng	186.5 g
jú hóng	橘紅		5 liǎng	186.5 g
bái fú líng	白茯苓		3 liǎng	111.9 g
gān cǎo	甘草	mix-fried with honey	1.5 liǎng	55.95 g

Usually cooked with ginger 薑 and wū méi 烏梅.

Tán's additions

xiāng fù	香附		1 qián	3.73 g
shén qū	神麴		1 qián	3.73 g
shā rén	砂仁		1 qián	3.73 g
cāng zhú	蒼朮		1 qián	3.73 g
hòu pǔ	厚朴		1 qián	3.73 g
chái hú	柴胡		1 qián	3.73 g
mù xiāng	木香		3 fēn	1.12 g

---

59. For example in *Jiā Yòu Bǔ Zhù Shén Nóng Běn Cǎo* 《 嘉祐補註神農本草 》 (published in 1060, *Sòng*). This association was still present in Tán's time as the passage from *Jiā Yòu Bǔ Zhù Shén Nóng Běn Cǎo* was recopied in *Běn Cǎo Gāng Mù* (published in 1597, *Míng*).

After the patient gave birth, she was still sick with an acute relapse of *nüè*-malarial dysentery and was given *Sì Wù Tāng* with two different sets of modification. Postpartum women were and still are commonly treated for blood deficiency and/or blood stasis, so *Sì Wù Tāng* is a logical base for a post-partum formula.

Case 12b
四物湯
Sì Wù Tāng (from *Jú Fāng*)
Decoction of Four Substances

dāng guī	當歸	
chuān xiōng	川芎	
bái sháo	白芍	
shú dì huáng	熟地黃	
		Tán's additions
xiāng fù	香附	
shén qū	神麴	dry-fried
shā rén	砂仁	
cāng zhú	蒼朮	
hòu pǔ	厚朴	
bái zhú	白朮	
chén pí	陳皮	
hēi gān jiāng	黑乾薑	removed in the next modification
xuán hú suǒ	玄胡索	removed in the next modification
cǎo guǒ	草菓	removed in the next modification

Besides supplementing and moving blood, the emphasis is on regulating qì, transforming dampness, and warming the middle *jiāo*.

After the patient was a little better, the formula was modified to:

Case 12c
四物湯
Sì Wù Tāng (from Jú Fāng)
Decoction of Four Substances

dāng guī	當歸	
chuān xiōng	川芎	
bái sháo	白芍	
shú dì huáng	熟地黃	
		Tán's additions
xiāng fù	香附	
shén qū	神麴	dry-fried
shā rén	砂仁	
cāng zhú	蒼朮	
hòu pǔ	厚朴	
bái zhú	白朮	
chén pí	陳皮	changed dose
rén shēn	人參	added to previous formula
mù xiāng	木香	added to previous formula
fú líng	茯苓	added to previous formula

Xiāng fù, shén qū, shā rén, cāng zhú, and *hòu pǔ* were included in the three formulas up until this point. The modifications from all three versions are similar to the ingredients of *Xiāng Shā Liù Jūn Zǐ Tāng* 香砂六君子湯 or *Xiāng Shā Yǎng Wèi Tāng* 香砂養胃湯, both of which harmonize the spleen and stomach when cold and damp are present in a deficient patient. We also have three of the main herbs from *Píng Wèi Sǎn* 平胃散.

Finally she took *Méng Jiāng Huáng Lián Wán* (from *Zhāi Xuán Fāng* - lost). This version of the formula is from Volume 4 of *Jì Shēng Fāng*.[60]

---

60. *Jì Shēng Fāng* 《濟生方》 is also known as *Yán Shì Jì Shēng Fāng* 《嚴氏濟生方》. It was written by Yán Yònghé 嚴用和 and published in 1253 (*Sòng*). The name of this formula is sometimes written as *Jiā Jiāng Huáng Lián Wán* 家薑黃連丸 or *Gān Jiāng Huáng Lián Wán* 乾薑黃連丸. The reason for calling it *Méng Jiāng* is uncertain, but in any case it refers to dried ginger.

蒙薑黃連丸

Méng Jiāng Huáng Lián Wán (from *Jì Shēng Fāng*)

Dried Ginger and Huáng Lián Pill

gān jiāng	乾薑	quick-fried	1 liǎng	37.3 g
huáng lián	黃連	remove the fine hairs	1 liǎng	37.3 g
suō shā rén	縮砂仁	dry-fried	1 liǎng	37.3 g
xiōng qióng	芎藭	mix-fried with honey	1 liǎng	37.3 g
ē jiāo	阿膠	filed, stir-fried in clam shell powder	1 liǎng	37.3 g
bái zhú	白朮		1 liǎng	37.3 g
rǔ xiāng	乳香	ground separately	3 qián	11.2 g
zhǐ qiào	枳殼	remove the pulp, dry-fry	0.5 liǎng	18.65 g

Powder the above, add a little vinegar together with three salted plums (remove the flesh), pestle it and make it into pills the size of *wú tóng zǐ* 梧桐子 (about 0.6-0.9 centimeters in diameter). Each dose is 40 pills. Taken as needed.

- Swallow them with a decoction of *gān jiāng* for white dysentery.
- Swallow them with a decoction of *gān cǎo* for red dysentery.
- Swallow them with a decoction of *gān jiāng* and *gān cǎo* for red and white dysentery.

This treats damage to the spleen by cold foods in pregnant women, or acrid and sour foods damaging the stomach, unregulated sensations of cold and heat, disquieted fetal qì, stagnant qì and congealed blood, intermittent red and white dysentery, intestinal rumbling, tenesmus, and pain in the rectum.

Case 13: Chronic Vomiting

一婦人，年五十二歲，患翻胃嘔吐，每日止飲酒幾甌，如見
米粒即嘔去，如是者一年，羸瘦太甚，身如死形。遂以火灸
五穴。

A 52 year old woman suffered an upset stomach with vomiting. Each day she only drank a few cups of liquor. She vomited if she even saw a grain of rice. She was this way for a year and became extremely emaciated; her body was like a corpse. I then used fire moxibustion on five points:

Shàng Wǎn (Rèn 13)	上脘	single point
Zhōng Wǎn (Rèn 12)	中脘	single point
Xià Wǎn (Rèn 10)	下脘	single point
Shí Guān (non-channel)	食關	bilateral point

初上艾火即爆去，比他人甚異；次又速粧艾炷，亦就爆去；
第三次方得火力，回家吃蝦羹一碗。又吃鮮魚粥一盞，即不
吐。

When I initially used mugwort fire, it burst into flames and went out, quite different than in other people. The next visit, I then quickly put mugwort cones on her, and again they burst into flames and went out right away. The third time, she returned home after obtaining the power of fire and ate a bowl of shrimp soup. She also ate a cup of fresh fish porridge and did not vomit.

次日二更，復嘔尤甚，見有一物將水盆漾之，天明視之，乃
一匾蟲也，長五寸濶一寸。許後服和胃白朮丸一料，飲食漸
加，形貌如常，遂獲痊安。

The next day during the second watch (around 9 to 11 p.m.), she vomited again and it was especially severe. Something could be seen making ripples in the water of the basin [where she vomited]. It was inspected at dawn and was a flatworm,[61] five cùn long and one cùn wide. A little later she took a batch of *Hé Wèi Bái Zhú Wán*. Her drinking and eating gradually increased, her appearance returned to normal, and she then was able to recover and regain her health.

Notes on Case 13

The Disease: *Fān wèi* 翻胃, here translated as upset stomach, can mean dysphagia, but more often symptoms include distention and fullness after eating, vomiting a long time after eating, undigested food in the vomit, and symptoms of deficiency coldness.

Perhaps a fair question to ask is whether she was simply an alcoholic. People did not usually drink plain water in ancient China as it was often unsafe. She might have selected boiled water, tea, or thin rice soup instead. However, it is common that people with parasites want specific foods, so perhaps it was the worm that was alcoholic, not the woman. The fact that she recovered later indicates that the desire for alcohol was related to her condition and was not alcoholism.

Treatment: Because this woman had been vomiting for a long time, she was so weak that she could not initially drink herbs. Therefore, Tán decided to treat with moxibustion. The burning moxa cones acted in a strange way on this patient. The implication is that this was related to the worms, which sometimes were seen as having supernatural powers in ancient culture. All of the moxibustion points were over the region where the worm resided. The moxibustion treatment successfully drove the worm out and the patient was able to recover.

In the section on phlegm in Volume 2 of *Dān Xī Zhì Fǎ Xīn Yào*, it discusses vomiting as a method of treating phegm disorders. After discussing various herbal strategies, it says "The shrimp broth vomiting method is also good."[62] The book never explains the details of this method. Could the

---

61. 匾蟲 is more commonly written 扁蟲. Both are pronounced *biǎn chóng*. This category includes flukes and tapeworms.
62. 蝦汁吐法亦好 。《丹溪治法心要 》

shrimp soup this woman had the previous day have contributed to this more therapeutic form of vomiting?

For discussion of the moxibustion treatment and *Hé Wèi Bái Zhú Wán* (or *Bái Zhú Hé Wèi Wán*), which treats stomach qì deficiency, see Case 10. For the moxibustion point Shí Guān, see Case 11.

Case 14: Lotus Leaf Lichen Wind Rash

一婦人，年二十三歲，患荷葉癬風。先與防風通聖散（出《袖珍方》），後與

A 23 year old woman suffered lotus leaf lichen wind. First I gave her *Fáng Fēng Tōng Shèng Săn* (from *Xiù Zhēn Fāng*). Afterwards I gave her

běi táo tóu	北桃頭
yáng tóu	楊頭
huáng jīng	黃荊
gŏu qĭ	枸杞
chūn shù	椿樹
fēi gŭ shēng fán	飛鹽生礬
jīn yín huā	金銀花
dòng shù gēn	楝樹根
zào jiăo	皂角

每晚洗一次。

Wash in it once each evening.

又莒茹散合六神散（俱出《摘玄方》），浴後用醋調前藥，以茄子擦上，如無茄子，用生薑擦。兩箇月即愈。

In another visit I gave her *Jŭ Rú Săn* and *Liù Shén Săn* (both from *Zhāi Xuán Fāng*). After washing [in the formula from the previous paragraph], mix the above herbs [*Jŭ Rú Săn* and *Liù Shén Săn*] with vinegar; use eggplant (*qié zĭ*) to rub [the vinegar mixture on the affected region]; if you don't have eggplant, rub with fresh ginger. She recovered in two months.

Notes on Case 14

The Disease: What is lotus leaf lichen wind (*hé yè xuăn fēng* 荷葉癬風)? Lichen (*xuăn*) is a skin condition characterized by scaling, itching, discharge, and elevation. There are many types, often named by their appearance: coin lichen, oxhide lichen, peach blossom lichen, pine bark lichen, etc. At this point, the details of lotus leaf lichen are unknown, but something in its appearance probably resembles a lotus leaf. The word *wind* is included as the etiology.

Treatment: This woman had a skin condition due to wind. She was given a formula named *Fáng Fēng Tōng Shèng Săn* from *Xiù Zhēn Fāng* to take internally.[63] Since no complete copy of *Xiù Zhēn Fāng* is available, here is the recipe from *Huáng Dì Sù Wèn Xuān Míng Lùn Fāng*:[64]

防風通聖散
Fáng Fēng Tōng Shèng Săn
(from *Huáng Dì Sù Wèn Xuān Míng Lùn Fāng*)
Fáng Fēng Powder to Communicate with the Sages

fáng fēng	防風		0.5 liăng	18.65 g
chuān xiōng	川芎		0.5 liăng	18.65 g
dāng guī	當歸		0.5 liăng	18.65 g

63. *Fáng Fēng Tōng Shèng Săn* is mentioned a few times for treating certain skin disorders in *Dān Xī Zhì Fă Xīn Yào* and *Dān Xī Xīn Fă* but the formula is never given. For example, Volume 6 of *Dān Xī Zhì Fă Xīn Yào* says, "For sores located in the upper body, Tōng Shèng Săn is often taken. 瘡在上多服通神散 。" Tán favored the formulas and treatment methods of Zhū Dānxī.

64. *Huáng Dì Sù Wèn Xuān Míng Lùn Fāng* 《 黃帝素問宣明論方 》 was written by Liú Wánsù 劉完素 and published in 1172 (*Jīn* dynasty).

sháo yào	芍藥		0.5 liǎng	18.65 g
dà huáng	大黃	processed with liquor	0.5 liǎng	18.65 g
bò hé	薄荷		0.5 liǎng	18.65 g
má huáng	麻黃		0.5 liǎng	18.65 g
lián qiáo	連翹		0.5 liǎng	18.65 g
máng xiāo	芒消		0.5 liǎng	18.65 g
shí gāo	石膏		1 liǎng	37.3 g
huáng qín	黃芩		1 liǎng	37.3 g
jié gěng	桔梗		1 liǎng	37.3 g
huá shí	滑石		3 liǎng	111.9 g
gān cǎo	甘草		2 liǎng	74.6 g
jīng jiè	荊芥		1 fēn	0.37 g
bái zhú	白朮		1 fēn	0.37 g
zhī zǐ	梔子		1 fēn	0.37 g

Powder the above. Each dose is 2 *qián* (7.46 grams) boiled in a big cup of water with three slices of ginger until 60% of the original volume. Take warm.

This formula treats excess heat that is simultaneously located in the interior and the exterior. Even though it contains a number of warm and hot herbs, the overall balance is quite cooling. *Má huáng* and *fáng fēng* release the exterior wind while *dà huáng* and *máng xiāo* eliminate internal heat through a bowel movement. *Dāng guī* and *sháo yào* supplement and regulate the blood, which is useful in wind-induced skin conditions. Historically this formula has been recommended for various types of rashes so its use in this case is not unusual.

Besides this, the patient was given an external wash. After decocting the wash, the patient should bathe the affected site in the liquid. Then she should scrub the region with a combination of two powders: *Jǔ Rú Sǎn* and *Liù Shén Sǎn*, mixed with vinegar. She should use a slice of eggplant or ginger to rub the vinegared powder into the affected site.

Both of these formulas originated from *Zhāi Xuán Fāng*, a book that is no longer extant. Since the book no longer exists, we must become medical detectives. No formula comes up in an internet search for *Jǔ Rú Sǎn* 莒茹

散. However, we can find *Lǚ Rú Sǎn* 閭茹散. It is likely that the first character in *Miscellaneous Records* was written incorrectly. The actual name of the formula is probably *Lǚ Rú Sǎn* 閭茹散, not *Jǔ Rú Sǎn* 莒茹散. *Jǔ* 莒 and *lǚ* 閭 look quite similar so *jǔ* 莒 is likely to be a 'misspelling' of *lǚ* 閭.

There are quite a few formulas named *Lǚ Rú Sǎn*, but only two are applied externally for rashes and similar disorders.

閭茹散

Lǚ Rú Sǎn (from Volume 13 of *Wèi Shēng Bǎo Jiàn**)
Lǚ Rú Powder

shuǐ yín	水銀		1 qián	3.73 g
hǎo chá	好茶		2 qián	7.46 g
lǚ rú	閭茹		3 qián	11.2 g
qīng fěn	輕粉		a small amount	

Make the above into a fine powder. Each time spread an appropriate amount mixed with oil on the affected site.

It treats scabby sores or scabies (*jiè*) that do not recover for years. It kills worms (*chóng*) and stops itching. †

**Wèi Shēng Bǎo Jiàn* 《 衛生寶鑑 》 was written by Luó Tiānyì 羅天益 and was published in 1343 (*Yuán*).

† *Shuǐ yín* is mercury and *qīng fěn* is a mercury compound, so this formula is not recommended for use today.

Lǐ Shízhēn's *Běn Cǎo Gāng Mù* writes the name of the herb as *lǚ rú* 藺茹 and gives a small recipe that is similar to the above: "For scabby sores [or scabies] with itching: Add some *qīng fěn* to powdered *lǚ rú* and mix it with sesame oil. From *Duō Néng Bǐ Shì*"[65, 66]

The other possibility is this:

---

65. *Duō Néng Bǐ Shì* 《 多能鄙事 》 is a twelve volume book that was written at the beginning of the *Míng* dynasty. Its author was Liú Jī 劉基 (1311-1375). While *Běn Cǎo Gāng Mù* was published in 1597, later than *Tán*'s book, the source of this small formula existed during *Tán*'s time.

66. 疥瘡瘙癢：藺茹末，入輕粉，香油調之 。《 多能鄙事 》 from 李時珍 《 本草綱目 》.

閭茹散
Lǘ Rú Sǎn (from Volume 90 of Tàipíng Shèng Huì Fāng*)
Lǘ Rú Powder

lǘ rú	閭茹		1 liǎng	37.3 g
sāng piāo shāo	桑螵蛸		1 liǎng	37.3 g
dì lóng	地龍		1 liǎng	37.3 g
rǔ xiāng	乳香		1 liǎng	37.3 g
huáng dān	黃丹		1 liǎng	37.3 g
huáng bǎi	黃柏	finely ground	1 liǎng	37.3 g
shè xiāng	麝香	finely ground	1 liǎng	37.3 g
nuò mǐ fěn	糯米粉		1 liǎng	37.3 g
nì fěn	膩粉		1 liǎng	37.3 g

Make the above into a fine powder. Each time, mix with well water and granulated sugar, and then apply it to the affected site.

For pediatric malign sores that last for a long time without recovery. [†]

*Tàipíng Shèng Huì Fāng 《太平圣惠方》 (992, Sòng) was edited by Wáng Huáiyǐn 王怀隐 et al.

[†] While this is a pediatric formula, it is possible that it was used on adults as well. Like the other formula with the same name, we are unlikely to use it today as *huáng dān* is red lead. *Nì fěn* is crystal mercurous chloride powder. *Shè xiāng* is expensive and there are ethical concerns about the treatment of the animals, although synthetic *shè xiāng* is available.

Jǔ Rú Sǎn (Lǘ Rú Sǎn) rubbed in with eggplant is also used in the next case and in Case 20.

There are also a number of formulas named *Liù Shén Sǎn* 六神散. Most of them are used internally. Only this one is used externally: *Liù Shén Sǎn* from Volume 16 of *Gǔ Jīn Yī Jiàn*[67]:

---

67. *Gǔ Jīn Yī Jiàn* 《古今醫鑑》 was written by Gōng Xìn 龔信, *Míng* dynasty.

六神散
Liù Shén Sǎn (from Volume 16 of *Gǔ Jīn Yī Jiàn*)
Six Spirits Powder

chuān wū	川烏	Use equal portions of each. On the day of Duānwǔ,* select the herbs and powder them. Each time, use a little bit. First smear saliva on the affected site, then rub it with the herbs.
cǎo wū	草烏	
nán xīng	南星	
bàn xià	半夏	Treats skin problems from scorpions (xiē máo 蠍蝥) and blister beetles (bān máo 斑蝥).
bái zhǐ	白芷	
shí chāng pú	石菖蒲	nine 1-cùn pieces

* Duānwǔ 端午 is the fifth day of the fifth lunar month, and occurs near the summer solstice. It is also the day of the Dragon Boat Festival and a day to take precautions against toxic critters such as scorpions and snakes.

The indications of this formula are different than those of this case, although both involve external medicine. It is possible that this is not the same formula Tán used, or maybe the formula took on expanded indications.

Xuǎn-lichens are scaly and itchy. Volume 6 of *Dān Xī Zhì Fǎ Xīn Yào* gives some different powdered formulas for external application to treat *xuǎn*-lichens. The procedure is generally this: Scrape the affected region to open it up. Mix the powdered formula with with vinegar and rub it in or apply it. This is similar to the procedure described by Tán.

As for the eggplant, both *Běn Cǎo Gāng Mù* and *Zhū Dānxī* (in *Běn Cǎo Yǎn Yì Bǔ Yí*《本草衍義補遺》) describe the topical use of various parts of the eggplant for treating sores and other skin conditions.

In any case, Tán gave the patient a decoction for internal use, as well as a wash and a scrub for external use.

Case 15: Postpartum Wind Itching

一婦人，年一十五歲，患滿面耳項風癢，不可當。詢其故，
昔日產後所得。某謂產後見風太早，氣血俱虛，其風乘虛，
而得於皮膚之間，似馬蟻，淫癢不可當。與補中益氣湯，
加：

A 15 year old woman suffered unbearable wind itching over her entire face,
ears, and nape. I inquired as to the reason; it began in the past after giving birth.
I said it was exposure to wind too soon after giving birth. Her qì and blood were
both deficient; the wind took advantage of the deficiency and got between the
layers of the skin. It felt like ants (*mǎ yǐ*) [crawling]; the oozing itch was unbearable. I gave her *Bǔ Zhōng Yì Qì Tāng*, adding:

shēng dì	生地	1 qián	3.73 g
xiāng fù	香附	2 qián	7.46 g

煎服。又付洗藥：

Decoct and take it. I also gave her an herbal wash:

zào jiǎo	皂角	4 liǎng	149.2 g
cāng zhú	蒼朮	4 liǎng	149.2 g

右水六碗，煎成膏，每朝洗面用一匙。又與莒茹散，茄子
擦，半月而愈。

Decoct the above in six bowls of water until it becomes concentrated. Each
morning wash the face using a soup-spoonful. I also gave her *Jǔ Rú Sǎn* (*Lǚ Rú
Sǎn* 閭茹散) to rub with eggplant (*qié zi*). She recovered in half a month.

Notes on Case 15

The Patient: This 15 year old is called a woman as she is already married and has had a baby. While this seems wrong today, it was a common age for marriage at the time. In fact, if a woman over the age of 15 is referred to as a girl in these cases, it probably implies that her disease has made her unmarriageable.

The Disease: This is another case of wind taking advantage of postpartum deficiency. It manifested as a skin condition, similar to Case 9. Zhū Dānxī wrote in *Dān Xī Zhì Fǎ Xīn Yào*, "In deficiency itching, blood is not abundant in the spaces between the flesh so it results in itching."[68]

Treatment: To fill in the empty space between the layers of the skin, Tán prescribed a formula that supplements post-heaven qì and blood. For *Bǔ Zhōng Yì Qì Tāng*, see Case 3. This formula supplemented her deficiency, the root of the itching. The added herbs (*shēng dì* and *xiāng fù*) cool and move the blood.

For *Jǔ Rú Sǎn* (*Lǔ Rú Sǎn* 閭茹散), see the previous case.

This woman was also given an herbal face wash of *zào jiǎo* and *cāng zhú*. *Zào jiǎo* is used externally or internally for many skin conditions. Zhū Dānxī (in *Běn Cǎo Yǎn Yì Bǔ Yì*) says it treats abscesses that have already ulcerated and guide a formula to the site of the abscess. It is also used for sores and lichens. *Běn Cǎo Gāng Mù* says *zào jiǎo* treats abscesses, malign sores, and kills *chóng*-bugs. *Cāng zhú* dries dampness.

---

68. 虛癢，血不榮肌腠，所以癢也 。朱丹溪《 丹溪治法心要 · 卷一 · 癩風 》

Case 16: Scrofula 2

一使女，年一十五歲，患瘰癧，兩頸有三十餘腫塊。每遇勞
碌、夏天大發寒熱，塊漸大。某與灸十六穴，腫塊遂消，後
不再發。隔一年後，曾食河豚毒物，亦不再發。

A 15 year old housemaid suffered scrofula sores with more than thirty swollen lumps on both sides of her neck. Whenever she was taxed from toil or in the summertime, chills and fever erupted and the lumps gradually enlarged. I gave her moxibustion on sixteen points [see below] and the swollen lumps then dissipated. They did not erupt again afterwards. A year later, she ate pufferfish (*hé tún*), which is a toxic thing, but they did not erupt again.

Yì Fēng (SJ 17)	醫風	bilateral point
Jiān Jǐng (GB 21)	肩井	bilateral point
Zhǒu Jiān (non-channel)	肘尖	bilateral point
Tiān Jǐng (SJ 10)	天井	bilateral point
Shǒu Sān Lǐ (LI 10)	手三里	bilateral point
Jiān Shǐ (PC 5)	間使	bilateral point
Nèi Guān (PC 6)	內關	bilateral point
Jué Gǔ (GB 39)	絕骨	bilateral point

Notes on Case 16

The Patient: Housemaid (*shǐ nǚ* 使女) could also be translated as female servant. The term does not specify whether she is married or not. Another housemaid is a patient in Case 19.

The Treatment: This is another case of scrofula. For discussion of the moxibustion treatment, see Case 5. The treatment was so successful that even when the patient had other health challenges later, the scrofula did not return.

Case 17: Insomnia

一富家老婦，年六十九歲，患氣虛痰火，全夜不睡，日中神思倦怠，諸藥不効。病及二年，右手寸關二部脈甚洪大，左手心脈大虛。詢其病原，乃因夫急症而故，痛極哭傷，遂得此症。

An older woman from a wealthy family, 69 years of age, suffered qì deficiency and phlegm fire. She could not sleep the entire night. At midday her mental state (*shén sī*) was tired and sluggish. Various medicines did not give results and the disease had lasted for two years. Both her right *cùn* and *guān* pulses were extremely surging and large; her heart pulse on the left was large but deficient. I inquired as to the source of the disease; it was because her husband had an acute ailment and had died; her pain was extreme with damage from weeping and then this ailment occurred.

某早晨用人參膏（出《摘玄方》）。日中用煎藥八物湯（出《丹溪方》）加：

I had her use *Rén Shēn Gāo* (from *Zhāi Xuán Fāng*) in the early morning. At midday she used a decoction of *Bā Wù Tāng* (from *Dān Xī Fāng*) adding:

dried shān yào	乾山藥	1 qián	3.73 g
suān zǎo rén	酸棗仁	1 qián	3.73 g
chén shā	辰砂	5 fēn	1.87 g
pú huáng	蒲黃	3 fēn	1.12 g
mù tōng	木通	7 fēn	2.61 g
yuǎn zhì	遠志	1 qián	3.73 g

水二鍾，薑三片，煎服。

Decoct in two cups of water with three slices of ginger and take it.

晚用琥珀鎮心丸（ 出《 丹溪方 》 ） 。

In the evenings she used *Hǔ Pò Zhèn Xīn Wán* (from *Dān Xī Fāng*).

至三更用清氣化痰丸（ 出《 摘玄方 》 ） 。

At the third watch (11p.m to 1 a.m), she used *Qīng Qì Huà Tán Wán* (from *Zhāi Xuán Fāng*).

不三月其症遂愈，後甚肥壯，壽至八十歲而終 。

Her ailment recovered in less than three months. Afterwards she was quite stout and strong, living until she was eighty years old and then passing on.

Notes on Case 17

The Disease: The oldest use of the term *damage from weeping* (*kū shāng* 哭傷) seems to be in the *Jiù Táng Shū* 《 舊唐書 》 (Old Táng History) where it describes a mother who has learned of her son's death. The first medical book in which these words appear together is probably *Shèng Jì Zǒng Lù* from the *Sòng* dynasty, but there it was simply a phrase, not an actual medical term. It reads "due to sorrowful weeping that damages the qì."[69] This is a similar idea but is not really a medical term.[70] In Tán's book, damage from weeping is found in this and the next case.

The patient was an older woman with fire that caused insomnia. Because of phlegm and lack of sleep, she was sluggish at noon. The right pulses showed excess and heat in the lungs/large intestine and spleen/stomach positions: the spleen makes phlegm while the lungs store it and the yáng-míng organs were hot. This heat and the excess condition of phlegm were reflected in the pulses on the right.

---

69. 因哀哭傷氣《 聖濟總錄 》 (Volume 116).
70. Thanks to Stephen Boyanton for the background on this term.

At the same time, the heart pulse was large and deficient. This reflected qì deficiency of the heart. Perhaps spleen qì was also deficient but the spleen/stomach pulse reflected the yángmíng heat instead, showing the more acute disorder.

Treatment: This patient received four formulas to be taken at four different times of the day.

Rén Shēn Gāo comes from a case study in an appended note to *Dān Xī Xīn Fǎ*. It consists of one ingredient: *rén shēn*. *Rén Shēn Gāo* returns original (*yuán* 元) qì. Zhū Dānxī used it for a patient who lost consciousness due to collapse of yáng. While he was waiting for the *rén shēn* to be boiled down to a thick paste, Zhū applied moxibustion at Qì Hǎi (Rèn 6). The patient recovered. In Tán's Case 17, the situation is not as acute, but Tán used this formula in the morning to arouse yáng so the patient would have better consciousness in the daytime.

At noon, the patient was given *Bā Wù Tāng* (see Case 1) to supplement qì and blood with added herbs to calm the spirit. In the daytime, Tán used formulas to strengthen and supplement. Even though the woman was sluggish, she used herbs to calm the spirit so the supplementation would not cause agitation. Since the disease was brought about by emotions, it is likely that Tán did not want to stir up more turmoil.

八物湯

Bā Wù Tāng

Decoction of Eight Substances

also known as *Bā Zhēn Tāng* 八珍湯 (Decoction of Eight Precious Ingredients)

四君子湯

Sì Jūn Zǐ Tāng

Decoction of Four Gentlemen

rén shēn	人參	remove the stem
bái zhú	白朮	
fú líng	茯苓	remove the peel
gān cǎo	甘草	honey-fried

四物湯
Sì Wù Tāng
Decoction of Four Substances

dāng guī	當歸	remove the stem, soak in liquor, and stir-fry
chuān xiōng	川芎	
bái sháo yào	白芍藥	
shú gān dì huáng	熟乾地黃	sprinkled with liquor and steamed

Tán's additions

dried shān yào	乾山藥	
suān zǎo rén	酸棗仁	
chén shā	辰砂	
pú huáng	蒲黃	
mù tōng*	木通	
yuǎn zhì	遠志	

Decoct in two cups of water with three slices of ginger and take it.

* This herb is usually avoided today due to its aristolochic acid content.

Hǔ Pò Zhèn Xīn Wán was used in the afternoon. It originally came from Volume 5 of *Hé Shì Jì Shēng Lùn*. Not much is known about this book, although it was cited by other books.

琥珀鎮心丸
Hǔ Pò Zhèn Xīn Wán (from Volume 5 of *Hé Shì Jì Shēng Lùn*)
Hǔ Pò Pill to Settle the Heart

hǔ pò	琥珀		5 qián	18.65 g
lóng chǐ	龍齒	calcined, ground	the original did not	
chuān lián	川連	stir-fried with liquor	specify the amount of these three medicinals	
zhū shā	硃砂			
mài dōng	麥冬		1 liǎng	37.3 g
tiān zhú huáng	天竺黃		7 qián	26.11 g
xī jiǎo	犀角		unspecified	
líng yáng jiǎo	羚羊角	ground	6 qián	22.38 g
zǎo rén	棗仁		unspecified	
yuǎn zhì	遠志		unspecified	

fú shén	茯神	5 qián	18.65 g
shí chāng pú	石菖蒲	5 qián	18.65 g
shè xiāng	麝香	2 qián	7.46 g
niú huáng	牛黃	3 qián	11.2 g
zhēn zhū	珍珠	2 qián	7.46 g
xióng huáng	雄黃	5 qián	18.65 g
jīn bó	金箔	40 sheets (as a covering)	

Make into honey pills the size of *lóng yǎn* 龍眼.

This formula is used when *shén*-spirit and *zhì*-will lose their guard; for withdrawal, mania, or delirium.

Tán gave this formula in the evening, to calm the patient down so she could sleep at night. While not specifically stated in the case, she seems to have yángmíng heat. Yángmíng heat and phlegm affecting the heart are both major causes of mania or delirium. These symptoms probably showed up at night time. *Hǔ Pò Zhèn Xīn Wán* then would fit the circumstances.

Hǔ Pò Zhèn Xīn Wán is certainly not for vegetarians: six of its 16 or 17 ingredients come from animal sources. Two additional ingredients are mineral. The wrapping is metal (gold foil which was consumed with the pills). And even though *hǔ pò* comes from a tree resin, it is fossilized, so it hardly counts as a typical plant product. Today there are legal, ethical, or price issues with the following: *zhū shā* (not legal in some places for internal use due to potential toxicity), *xī jiǎo* (endangered), *shè xiāng* (price, animal cruelty), *niú huáng* and *jīn bó* (price), and *xióng huáng* (not for internal use due to toxicity). It is unlikely that this formula could be prescribed today.

Qīng Qì Huà Tán Wán was used around midnight. Here is *Qīng Qì Huà Tán Wán* from Volume 9 of *Dān Xī Xīn Fǎ Fù Yú* (An Appendix to *Dān Xī Xīn Fǎ*).[71]

---

71. *Dān Xī Xīn Fǎ Fù Yú* 《丹溪心法附餘》 (An Appendix to *Dān Xī Xīn Fǎ*) was published in 1536. This source was published later than Tán's book, but since it came from a Zhū Dānxī source, it is probably similar to what she used. Note that this formula is quite different from the one found in Bensky, which was taken from an even later source. Only four of the ingredients are the same.

清氣化痰丸
Qīng Qì Huà Tán Wán
(from Volume 9 of *Dān Xī Xīn Fǎ Fù Yú*)
Qì-Clearing Phlegm-Transforming Pill

bàn xià	半夏	wash in hot water 7 times	2 liǎng	74.6 g
chén pí	陳皮	remove the white	1.5 liǎng	55.95 g
fú líng	茯苓	remove the peel	1.5 liǎng	55.95 g
bò hé yè	薄荷葉		5 qián	18.65 g
jīng jiè suì	荊芥穗		5 qián	18.65 g
huáng qín	黃芩	soaked in liquor	1 liǎng	37.3 g
lián qiáo	連翹		1 liǎng	37.3 g
zhī zi rén	梔子仁	stir-fried	1 liǎng	37.3 g
jié gěng	桔梗	remove the stem	1 liǎng	37.3 g
gān cǎo	甘草	honey-fried	1 liǎng	37.3 g

Powder the above and make into pills the size of *wú tóng zǐ* 梧桐子 (about 0.6-0.9 centimeters in diameter) with a flour paste made with ginger juice and boiled water. Each dose is 50 pills, taken after eating and at bedtime. Clears the head and eyes, cools the diaphragm, transforms phlegm, and disinhibits qì.

This formula is an adaptation of *Èr Chén Tāng*, so it regulates qì and transforms phlegm and dampness. It also has quite a few herbs to clear heat in the upper body. This formula was given at midnight, to treat the root.

We could look at the treatment this way:

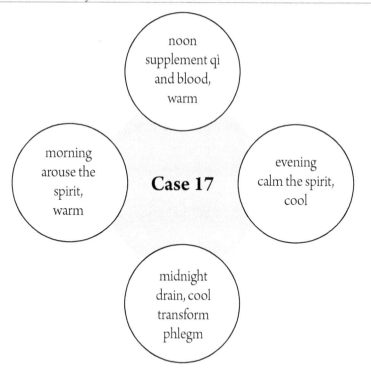

We can see that at dawn and dusk, the main thrust of the formulas was to adjust the spirit. At noon and midnight, the principle was to treat the main patterns. In the yáng times, warm and supplement; in the yín times, cool and drain.

The woman recovered and lived 11 more years.

Case 18: *Wěi*-Atrophy 1

一富家婦，年四十五歲，得患痿症一年，不能起床。聞人聲
響，即虛暈，或大便小便後，亦虛暈，兩手脈甚細弱，乃氣
血皆虛。又咳嗽，痰中見血。詢其故，先因有女身故，痛極
哭傷；不隔半年，其夫變故，又因哭傷加病，其婦性亦躁
急。某先用瓊玉膏，加：

A 45 year old woman from a wealthy household suffered a *wěi*-atrophy ailment for a year and was unable to get out of bed. When she heard the sound
of people talking, she experienced deficiency dizziness; she also sometimes experienced deficiency dizziness after defecation or urination. The pulses of both
hands were extremely thin and weak. This was deficiency of both qì and blood.
She also had a cough with blood in the sputum. I inquired as to the reason; the
first cause was her daughter dying, which was extremely painful so there was
damage from weeping. Not half a year had gone by when her husband had an
accident [or died]; damage from weeping again contributed to her disease. The
woman's nature was also quick-tempered and impatient.

I first used *Qióng Yù Gāo*, adding:

biǎn bǎi yè	匾栢葉	1 liǎng	37.3 g
bèi mǔ	貝母	1 liǎng	37.3 g

次用人參六君子湯（出《局方》）、四物湯，加：

I next used *Rén Shēn Liù Jūn Zǐ Tāng* (from *Jú Fāng*) and *Sì Wù Tāng*, adding:

huáng lián	黃連	1 qián	3.73 g
shān zhī rén	山梔仁	8 fēn	2.98 g
xiāng fù	香附	1 qián	3.73 g

臨睡與硃砂安神丸 。治之半月稍愈，三月後遂得起床 。

At bedtime, I gave her *Zhū Shā Ān Shén Wán*. I treated her for half a month and there was slight improvement; after three months, she was able to get out of bed.

Notes on Case 18

The Disease: This case has some similarities to the previous one. Both women were damaged by grief and weeping, but this case is pure deficiency while the previous one also suffered from phlegm fire. This case also has heat - the woman was quick-tempered and impatient, and all emotions, including grief, can lead to qì constraint over time. Qì constraint leads to heat, especially in the liver. When a hot liver stores blood, it heats up the blood. This apparently led to coughing of blood. However, based on the pulses, the main pathology was deficiency.

Treatment: Tán did not mention the source for *Qióng Yù Gāo* (which is also used in Case 26). It is from *Hóng Shì Jí Yàn Fāng*.[72]

瓊玉膏
Qióng Yù Gāo (from *Hóng Shì Jí Yàn Fāng*)
Beautiful Jade Syrup

rén shēn	人參		24 liǎng	895.2 g
bái fú líng	白茯苓		16 jīn	9548.8 g
shēng dì huáng	生地黃	pounded to make juice	48 liǎng	1790.4 g
honey	白蜜		10 jīn	5968 g

Powder the *rén shēn* and *fú líng*. Strain the honey through raw silk. Use the juice from *dì huáng*, but do not use iron materials in processing it; after juicing the *dì huáng*, dispose of the dregs. Put the ingredients together and blend evenly; seal them in silver, stoneware, or porcelain, and save it for when it is needed. Take two soup-spoonfuls each morning, dissolved in warm liquor; if the person does not drink liquor, dissolve it in hot water.

This formula enriches yīn, moistens dryness, boosts qì, and nourishes blood.

---

72. *Hóng Shì Jí Yàn Fāng* 《洪氏集驗方》 was written by Hóng Zūn 洪遵 and published in 1170 (*Sòng*).

Here, Tán added *biǎn bǎi yè* and *bèi mǔ* for cough with blood in sputum; no modifications were mentioned in Case 26.

Tán attributed *Rén Shēn Liù Jūn Zǐ Tāng* to *Jú Fāng* but while *Sì Jūn Zǐ Tāng* is in *Jú Fāng*, *Liù Jūn Zǐ Tāng* is not (at least not by that name). A bit of a mystery is why she called it *Rén Shēn Liù Jūn Zǐ Tāng* when *rén shēn* is already an ingredient of *Liù Jūn Zǐ Tāng*. One thought would be to emphasize that *dǎng shēn* was not to be substituted for *rén shēn*. However, it seems that *dǎng shēn* was not commonly used and did not replace *rén shēn* until later, in the *Qīng* dynasty. However, *rén shēn* was already becoming harder to get and more expensive in the *Míng* dynasty due to unsustainable use so perhaps *rén shēn* was added to the name of the formula to be sure the patient or pharmacy did not skimp on it.[73] Other possible reasons for including *rén shēn* in the name include: there could have been another formula by the same name that did not use *rén shēn* (unlikely), to emphasize the use of *rén shēn* enhances the importance of the formula, that it is a combination of *Rén Shēn Tāng* and *Liù Jūn Zǐ Tāng*, or that there is an increased dose of *rén shēn*. We have no answer to this question. *Rén Shēn Liù Jūn Zǐ Tāng* was also used in Case 26 without modifications.

Here is *Liù Jūn Zǐ Tāng* from Volume 4 of *Dān Xī Xīn Fǎ*:

六君子湯
Liù Jūn Zǐ Tāng (from Volume 4 of Dān Xī Xīn Fǎ)
Six Gentlemen Decoction

rén shēn	人參
bái zhú	白朮
fú líng	茯苓
gān cǎo	甘草
shā rén	砂仁
chén pí	陳皮

---

73. *Was the item used as Ren Shen in ancient times actually Dang Shen?* by Eric Brand, http://www.legendaryherbs.com/blog/110085/7891/ posted on 6/17/2012 and accessed on 1/11/2015. Thanks also to Eric Brand for his personal comments on this issue.

Boil in water with three slices of ginger and one piece of *dà zǎo*.
It harmonizes the spleen and stomach; for difficulty swallowing food and drink.

There is a note that another book uses *bàn xià* 半夏 instead of *shā rén*; today *bàn xià* is more commonly used. We do not know which herb Tán selected.

Tán added *Sì Wù Tāng* and other herbs, so here is the final formula:

Case 18

六君子湯
Liù Jūn Zǐ Tāng
Six Gentlemen Decoction

rén shēn	人參
bái zhú	白朮
fú líng	茯苓
gān cǎo	甘草
shā rén	砂仁
chén pí	陳皮

四物湯
Sì Wù Tāng
Decoction of Four Substances

dāng guī	當歸
chuān xiōng	川芎
bái sháo	白芍
shú dì huáng	熟地黃

Tán's additions

huáng lián	黃連
shān zhī rén	山梔仁
xiāng fù	香附

Note that we could also consider this *Bā Wù Tāng* (also known as *Bā Zhēn Tāng*; see Case 1) with additions, which would also be appropriate for the diagnosis of deficiency of both qì and blood. However, the dizziness and cough indicate that there is some phlegm-dampness present. Calling it *Liù Jūn Zǐ Tāng* tells us that Tán was thinking the phlegm-dampness was significant, not just the deficiency.

While insomnia was not mentioned, this woman was emotionally distressed. *Zhū Shā Ān Shén Wán* was given at night to calm the spirit and help *her to sleep. It not only calms the spirit, but because it cools blood in the* chest, this formula may help with the coughing of blood. Tán did not mention the source of this formula. It is from *Lán Shì Mì Cáng by* Lǐ Dōngyuán (*Jīn*).[74]

硃砂安神丸
Zhū Shā Ān Shén Wán (from *Lán Shì Mì Cáng*)
Zhū Shā Pill to Calm the Spirit

zhū shā*	硃砂		0.5 liǎng	18.65 g
huáng lián	黃連		6 qián	22.38 g
zhì gān cǎo	炙甘草		5.5 qián	20.52 g
shēng dì huáng	生地黃		2.5 qián	9.33 g
dāng guī	當歸		2.5 qián	9.33 g

Water grind the *zhū shā* separately until it is like dust, dry in the shade, and use it to coat the pills. Make the other herbs into a fine powder. Make into pills the size of a grain of millet. Each dose is 25 pills (about 2 grams), swallowed with saliva after meals.

Treats vexation and confusion of the heart with palpitations, sudden desire to vomit, chaotic qì in the chest and heat or fever. This is fire lurking in the blood above the diaphragm, and heavy herbs are needed to press down the yīn fire that is floating up. It also nourishes the upper *jiāo*.

* Zhū shā is not used internally today due to its potential for toxicity and its internal use may be illegal in some jurisdictions.

This was a chronic case and it took three months for the patient to improve.

---

74. *Lán Shì Mì Cáng* was written by Lǐ Dōngyuán (*Jīn*) 李東垣《 蘭室秘藏·卷下雜病門 》. It is also found in other books authored by Lǐ. He called it *Ān Shén Wán* 安神丸.

Case 19: Jaundice

一富家使女，年一十八歳，因患傷寒，病起三月後，勞碌大
發熱，遂成黃疸，即女勞疸。

Because an 18 year old housemaid of a wealthy family suffered from cold damage, three months later she was sick with with high fever due to taxation from toil. This developed into jaundice, meaning female taxation jaundice.

先用枸杞根（一把）搗汁大酒和服。

I first used *gǒu qǐ gēn* (one handful) pounded to make juice, mixed with great liquor, and gave it to her to take.

又用四苓湯（出《局方》），加

I also used *Sì Líng Tāng* (from *Jú Fāng*), adding:

bàn xià	半夏	1 qián	3.73 g
mù tōng	木通	7 fēn	2.61 g
shān zhī	山梔	8 fēn	2.98 g
dāng guī	當歸	1 qián	3.73 g
chuān xiōng	川芎	1 qián	3.73 g
dì huáng	地黃	1 qián	3.73 g
sháo yào	芍藥	1 qián	3.73 g
xiāng fù	香附	1 qián	3.73 g
huáng qín	黃芩	1 qián	3.73 g

水二鍾，薑三片，食後，煎服。數帖，即愈。

Decoct in two cups of water with three slices of ginger and take it after meals. She recovered after several packets.

Notes on Case 19

The Disease: *Nǚ láo dǎn* 女勞疸 translates literally as female taxation jaundice and was first discussed in *Jīn Guì Yào Lüè* 《金匱要略》. It is associated with bedroom taxation, drunkenness, and over-eating. Symptoms include jaundice, fever that is worse at dusk, aversion to cold, warm soles, urinary urgency, fullness of the lower abdomen, a dark forehead, and so forth. The treatment for it in *Jīn Guì Yào Lüè* is *Xiāo Shí Fán Shí Sǎn* 硝石礬石散 (although Tán used a different formula).

The term generally seems to refer to a man sexually wearing himself out (hence the *female* in this term) and then developing jaundice. Here the patient is a woman and the described etiology is excessive toil combined with cold damage. Perhap the *toil* is actually sexual excess – it is certainly possible that one of the men in the household was fond of her. In these cases Tán never explicitly mentioned sexual activity even when it seems to be relevant so "taxation from toil" may be a euphemism.

On the other hand, Tán may be using "female taxation jaundice" more literally - a woman who develops jaundice after working too hard. This is one of two cases that mentions cold damage, and the only time Tán prescribed a formula somewhat related to the works of Zhāng Zhòngjǐng (see below). Her emphasis was on the medicine developed in the *Sòng-Jīn-Yuán* period so her use of the term *female taxation jaundice* may not be the same as in *Jīn Guì Yào Lüè*.

Treatment: *Gǒu qǐ gēn* is an alternate name for *dì gǔ pí* 地骨皮. It clears heat in deficiency and taxation. She drank juice from the fresh root that was mixed with a special liquor. Great liquor (*dà jiǔ* 大酒) is the name of a special drink fermented in the winter and aged until summer. It was mentioned in the *Sòng* History (*Sòng Shǐ* 《宋史》). Perhaps this liquor is more cooling since it is made in winter. *Dà jiǔ* is also used in the next case.

There is no formula from *Jú Fāng* named *Sì Líng Tāng* or *Sì Líng Sǎn* although it does have *Wǔ Líng Sǎn*. Volume 2 of *Dān Xī Xīn Fǎ* says, "*Sì Líng*

Sǎn means *Wǔ Líng Sǎn* with the *guì* removed."[75] *Wǔ Líng Sǎn* consists of *zé xiè* 澤瀉, *zhū líng* 豬苓, *fú líng* 茯苓, *bái zhú* 白朮, and *guì zhī* 桂枝. With the *guì zhī* removed, later commentors tell us that the formula only percolates dampness and disinhibits water without warming yáng. This is appropriate as the patient had a high fever. Perhaps this formula was called a decoction (*tāng*) rather than a powder (*sǎn*) because of how it was to be prepared and perhaps it was misattributed. If this is correct, now the formula looks like this:

Case 19
四苓散
Sì Líng Sǎn (from Volume 2 of Dān Xī Xīn Fǎ)
Six Gentlemen Decoction

zé xiè	澤瀉	
zhū líng	豬苓	
fú líng	茯苓	
bái zhú	白朮	
		Tán's additions
bàn xià	半夏	
mù tōng	木通	
shān zhī	山梔	
dāng guī	當歸	These four make *Sì Wù Tāng*.
chuān xiōng	川芎	
dì huáng	地黃	
sháo yào	芍藥	
xiāng fù	香附	
huáng qín	黃芩	

Decocted with ginger.

This formula then promotes urination to drain the damp and clear the heat that caused jaundice. It also supplements blood and regulates qì.

---

75. 四苓散即五苓散內去桂 。《 丹溪心法 》

Case 20: Litchee Nose

一女子，年八歲，患荔枝鼻至十五歲，諸藥不効。先用搽藥
方莒茹散。又用煎藥（出《時先生方》）薑三片，煎服。

An eight year old girl suffered litchee (*lì zhī*) nose until she was fifteen. Various
medicines did not give results. I first used the topical herbal formula *Jǔ Rú Sǎn*
(*Lǘ Rú Sǎn* 閭茹散). In another visit I used an herbal decoction (from *Shí
Xiān Shēng Fāng*) boiled with three slices of ginger and taken.[76]

又用洗面藥（出《袖珍方》）。右為粗末分，作十帖，每帖
用水三升，煎五七沸，去粗，早晚洗面二次。

In another visit I used Face-Washing Herbs (*Xǐ Miàn Yào*) (from *Xiù Zhēn
Fāng*). Make the formula into a coarse powder and divide it into ten packets.
Each packet is used with three *shēng* of water and boiled five or seven rollings.
Remove the coarse parts and wash the face with it twice a day: morning and
evening.

又用何首烏丸（出《丹溪方》）：

In another visit I used *Hé Shǒu Wū Wán* (from *Dān Xī Fāng*):

hé shǒu wū	何首烏	5 jīn	2984 g
shēng dì huáng	生地黃	1 jīn	586.8 g
honey	白蜜	2 jīn	1193.6 g
dà jiǔ	大酒	unspecified	

勻和為丸，每日一二次，甘草湯下，七十丸。服盡即愈。

Mix evenly and make it into pills. Take them once or twice each day, swallowing seventy pills [each time] with a decoction of *gān cǎo*. She recovered after
taking them all.

---

76. There is probably something missing here. A decoction is mentioned but no name
for the formula or ingredients are given. Yet we are told to boil it with three slices of
ginger. The book, Mr. Shí's Formulas (*Shí Xiān Shēng Fāng*) is unknown.

Notes on Case 20

The Disease: Litchee (*lì zhī*) nose would be a big red bumpy nose appearing like a lichee, perhaps rosacea in biomedicine.

Treatment: For *Jǔ Rú Sǎn* (*Lǔ Rú Sǎn* 閭茹散), see Case 14.

Xǐ Miàn Yào is originally from *Lán Shì Mì Cáng* by Lǐ Dōngyuán.

洗面藥
Xǐ Miàn Yào (from Volume 3 of *Lán Shì Mì Cáng*)
Face-Washing Herbs
also called *Xǐ Miàn Sǎn* 洗面散 (Face-Washing Powder)

zào jiǎo	皂角	pound separately	3 jīn	1790.4 g
shēng má	好升麻	good quality	8 liǎng	298.4 g
chǔ shí zǐ	楮實子		5 liǎng	186.5 g
bái jí	白及	finely filed	1 liǎng	37.3 g
gān sōng	甘松		7 qián	26.11 g
suō shā	縮砂	with the skin	5 fēn	1.87 g
bái dīng xiāng	白丁香	gathered in the 12th lunar month	5 fēn	1.87 g
sān nài zǐ	三奈子		5 fēn	1.87 g
lǜ dòu	綠豆		8 gě	858.96 ml
nuò mǐ	糯米		1 shēng 2 gě	1288.44 ml

Make the above into a fine powder. Wash the face with it.
Removes skin, treats dry itching, removes grease, makes the skin and flesh smooth and moist. Treats freckles on the face, sores, acne, pimples, and the like.

Tán gave the recipe for *Hé Shǒu Wū Wán* in her text, saying it is a Zhū Dānxī formula but it is not found in *Dān Xī Zhì Fǎ Xīn Yào* or *Dān Xī Xīn Fǎ*. There are many different recipes for pills by this name found in an internet search, but none have the listed ingredients. Perhaps this is why Tán gave the recipe; it doesn't seem to be common. *Hé Shǒu Wū Wán* is also used in Case 23.

Case 21: Diaphragm Qì

一婦人，年五十六歲，得患隔氣半年，諸藥不効。某詢其
故，云因夫貴娶妾，憂忿成疾。又詢其曾服何藥，醫者任用
理氣之劑，多耗元氣，以致神思倦怠，飲食不進。某用生血
益元化痰之劑，灸：

A 56 year old woman suffered from *gé*-diaphragm qì[77] for half a year. Various
medicines did not give results. I inquired as to the reason; she said because her
high ranking husband took a concubine, sorrow and anger had developed into
illness. I then inquired about what medicine she had taken in the past; doctors
had employed prescriptions to rectify qì which consumed much of her original
qì. The result was that her mental state (*shén sī*) was tired and sluggish[78] and
she could not swallow drink and food. I used prescriptions to engender blood,
boost the origin, and transform phlegm, and I applied moxibustion to:

Shàng Wǎn (Rèn 13)	上脘	single point
Zhōng Wǎn (Rèn 12)	中脘	single point
Xià Wǎn (Rèn 10)	下脘	single point
Shí Guān (non-channel)	食關	bilateral point

服六味地黃丸（出《摘玄方》），煎藥，四物湯兼二陳湯，
加：

She took *Liù Wèi Dì Huáng Wán* (from *Zhāi Xuán Fāng*) and a decoction of *Sì
Wù Tāng* combined with *Èr Chén Tāng*, adding:

bái zhú	白朮	1 qián	3.73 g
xiāng fù	香附	1 qián	3.73 g
zhǐ shí	枳實	1 qián	3.73 g
cāng zhú	蒼朮	1 qián	3.73 g

---

77. 隔氣 (separation qì) is more correctly written as 膈氣 (diaphragm qì). Both are pronounced *gé qì*. The right part of the two *gé* characters is the same. 隔means to separate,
which is what the diaphragm (膈) does.
78. This should be written *juàn dài* 倦怠 but instead has *quán dài* 惓怠.

水二鍾，薑三片，煎服 。二十帖遂獲全愈 。

Decoct in two cups of water with three slices of ginger, and take it. After twenty packets, she was able to completely recover.

Notes on Case 21

The Disease: In *gé*-diaphragm qì, the region of the chest and diaphragm are obstructed (the throat is perhaps seen as separated from the stomach by the diaphragm) so it is hard to swallow. Dysphagia is one of the main symptoms and difficulty swallowing makes it difficult to eat (often leading to emaciation) and to take medicine.

The previous doctors had used herbs that were too harsh for this woman's condition, leaving her mentally dull and physically weaker. In addition, the emotional causes were still present.

Treatment: For the moxibustion treatment, please see the discussion in Case 10. Since this woman could not easily swallow medicine, moxibustion to treat the middle *jiāo* was a good option.

Tán wrote, "I used prescriptions to engender blood, boost the origin, and transform phlegm." She used *Sì Wù Tāng* to engender blood, *Liù Wèi Dì Huáng Wán* to boost the origin, and *Èr Chén Tāng* to transform phlegm.

While *Liù Wèi Dì Huáng Wán* is an older formula (originally penned by Qián Yǐ 錢乙 in the *Sòng* dynasty), let's take it from Volume 3 of *Dān Xī Xīn Fǎ*. There it is called *Jīn Guì Shèn Qì Wán* 金匱腎氣丸 but *Liù Wèi Dì Huáng Wán* is listed as an alternate name.

六味地黄丸
Liù Wèi Dì Huáng Wán (from Volume 3 of *Dān Xī Xīn Fǎ*)
Dì Huáng Pill with Six Ingredients

dried shān yào	干山藥	4 liǎng	149.2 g
shān zhū yú	山茱萸	4 liǎng	149.2 g
zé xiè	澤瀉	3 liǎng	111.9 g
mǔ dān pí	牡丹皮	3 liǎng	111.9 g
fú líng	茯苓	3 liǎng	111.9 g
shú dì huáng	熟地黃	8 liǎng	298.4 g

Powder the above and make honey pills the size of *wú zǐ* 梧子 (about 0.6-0.9 centimeters in diameter). Take 50 or 60 pills on an empty stomach with warm water. Treats emaciation, weakness, long term kidney qì deficiency, withered appearance, night sweating and fevers; all five *zàng*-organs are harmed.

Liù Wèi Dì Huáng Wán was originally written as a pediatric formula. It took a while for it to develop the uses and functions we give it today. The above is not too far off, though. Since this is how Zhū Dānxī saw it, it is probably how Tán understood it.

For *Sì Wù Tāng* and *Èr Chén Tāng*, see Case 6. The final formula comes out to this:

Case 21
四物湯
Sì Wù Tāng
Decoction of Four Substances

dāng guī	當歸
chuān xiōng	川芎
bái sháo	白芍
shú dì huáng	熟地黃

二陳湯
Èr Chén Tāng
Decoction of Two Aged Ingredients

bàn xià	半夏

jú hóng	橘紅
fú líng	茯苓
gān cǎo	甘草

Usually cooked with ginger and *wū méi* 烏梅.

Tán's additions

bái zhú	白朮
xiāng fù	香附
zhǐ shí	枳實
cāng zhú	蒼朮

Decocted with ginger.

It seems that the moxibustion was the only treatment focused on the diaphragm qì. The herbal treatment was directed at her deficiency patterns and the phlegm. These actions should help her weak body and her dull mental state.

Case 22: Postpartum Taxation

一婦人，年二十七歲，得患產後寒熱，將一年甚是憔瘦。又兼咳嗽將危，諸藥不効。某以產後勞傷，治之灸：

A 27 year old woman suffered [sensations of] heat and cold after giving birth; almost a year later she was extremely withered and emaciated. At the same time, she was also coughing and was near death. Various medicines did not give results. I took it as damage due to postpartum taxation and treated it with moxibustion:

Gāo Huāng (UB 43)	膏肓	bilateral point
Pí Shù (UB 20)	脾腧	bilateral point
Dà Zhuì (Dū 14)	大椎	single point
Sān Lǐ (ST 36)	三里	bilateral point

用調中益氣湯十帖（出《試效方》）。又用和胃白朮丸。又
與雄黃二兩，佩之胸前，鼻聞其氣則殺勞蟲。不一月其患遂
愈。

She used ten packets of *Tiáo Zhōng Yì Qì Tāng* (from *Shì Xiào Fāng*). In another
visit, she used *Hé Wèi Bái Zhú Wán*. I also gave her two *liǎng* (74.6 grams) of
xióng huáng to wear [as a sachet] on her chest; smelling its qì [aroma] kills consumption *chóng*-worms. In less than a month, her suffering recovered.

Notes on Case 22

Treatment: A similar moxibustion treatment is seen in Case 10 (the second moxibustion point formula there). The difference between this point
formula and the one in Case 10 is that here the lung's *shù* point is used
instead of the spleen's. It seems then that in deep deficiency, Tán combined
Dà Zhuì (Dū 14), Gāo Huāng (UB 43), and Zú Sān Lǐ (ST 36) with the
back *shù* point of the most depleted organ.

Tiáo Zhōng Yì Qì Tāng was attributed to *Shì Xiào Fāng*[79] but this formula is
originally from *Pí Wèi Lùn* by Lǐ Dōngyuán.

調中益氣湯
Tiáo Zhōng Yì Qì Tāng (from Pí Wèi Lùn)
Decoction to Regulate the Center and Boost Qì

huáng qí	黃芪		1 qián	3.73 g
rén shēn	人參	remove the stem	0.5 qián	1.87 g
zhì gān cǎo	炙甘草		0.5 qián	1.87 g
chén pí	陳皮		2 fēn	0.75 g
wǔ wèi zǐ	五味子			7 pcs
sháo yào	芍藥		3 fēn	1.12 g
bái zhú	白朮		5 fēn	1.87 g

79. The full name of the book is *Dōng Yuán Shì Xiào Fāng* 羅謙甫《東垣試效方》
by Luó Qiānfǔ, *Yuán*, a disciple of Lǐ Dōngyuán 李東垣.

dāng guī	當歸	5 fēn	1.87 g
shēng má	升麻	2 fēn	0.75 g
chái hú	柴胡	2 fēn	0.75 g

Break the above into small bits. This is one dose. Boil in 2 cups of water down to 1 cup. Remove the dregs. Take warm before meals.
Treats spleen-stomach damage due to hunger, overeating, and taxation.

For *Hé Wèi Bái Zhú Wán*, see Case 10. It treats stomach qì deficiency and harmonizes the center, rectifies qì, disperses phlegm, removes dampness, harmonizes the spleen and stomach, and enables one to eat and drink.

These two formulas helped restore the patient's ability to replenish post-heaven qì.

The Disease: Consumption worms (*láo chóng* 勞蟲) would more literally be translated as *taxation worms*. Taxation 勞 and consumption 癆 are both pronounced *láo*. In writing, consumption is the character for taxation plus the disease radical. Sometimes the character taxation 勞 is substituted for consumption 癆. Consumption, in many cases, is the equivalent of tuberculosis in Western medicine. Two of the main symptoms are emaciation and cough, both of which occured in this patient. In ancient times, consumption was often attributed to *chóng*-worms. The word *chóng* 蟲 has a much broader range of meaning then *worms* in English. It can include snakes, bugs, reptiles, and the like (creepy-crawlies), as well as some invisible disease-causing entities.

Treatment: An interesting method of treatment sometimes found in old books is to use a sachet of herbs, usually attached to the clothing or hung on a string around the neck. The patient passively breathes in its aroma all day long and is usually told to sniff it occasionally. In addition, wearing it near points such as Dàn Zhōng (Ren 17) may also have an influence. The herbs placed in the sachet are selected according to the condition to be treated. Tán said that smelling *xióng huáng* (realgar) kills consumption *chóng*-worms. Lǐ Shízhēn reported in Volume 9 of *Běn Cǎo Gāng Mù* that *xióng huáng*, a mineral, kills consumption worms (using the same words as Tán: *láo chóng* 勞蟲).

Case 23: Infertility

一婦人，三十二歲，生四胎後，十年不生。因無子，甚是憂悶。某詢其故，乃因夫不時宿娼，偶因經事至，大鬧乘時。多耗氣血，遂成白淋，小腹冷痛。

A 32 year old woman had given birth four times, but in [the following] ten years she had not given birth again. Because she had no son, she was extremely depressed. I inquired as to the reason [for her condition]; it was because her husband frequently spent the night with female performers. Whenever her menstrual period arrived, she took advantage of the time to strongly vent her anger. Much of her qì and blood was consumed, and then it developed into white *lín*-dribbling. Her lower abdomen was cold and painful.

某思《脈訣》云：「崩中日久，為白帶；漏下之時，骨木枯」，即子宮虛冷以致，不能成胎。某與灸暖子宮。又《明堂鍼灸》云：鍼則絕產；灸之三遍令人生產。某取灸：

I considered what *Mài Jué*[80] says: "Flooding (*bēng*) over a long period of time becomes white [vaginal] *dài*-discharge; in times of spotting (*lòu*), the bones become like withered wood." The result is that the Child's Palace (*zǐ gōng* - the uterus) becomes deficient and cold, unable to produce a pregnancy. I gave her moxibustion to warm the Child's Palace. In addition, *Míng Táng Zhēn Jiǔ*[81] says that acupuncture cuts off childbearing but three complete applications of moxibustion enables a person to give birth. I selected the following for moxibustion:

Qì Hǎi (Rèn 6)	氣海	single point
Guān Yuán (Rèn 4)	關元	single point
Zhōng Jí (Rèn 3)	中極	single point
Qì Chōng (ST 30)	氣衝	bilateral point

---

80. *Mài Jué* 崔嘉言《脈訣》(Rhymed Songs of Pulse) was written by Cuī Jiāyán (*Sòng*).

81. See the discussion in the notes below.

服何首烏丸（ 出《 丹溪方 》 ），連灸三年，遂產一子 。

She took *Hé Shǒu Wū Wán* (from *Dān Xī Fāng*) and continuously received moxibustion for three years. She then gave birth to a son.

Notes on Case 23

The Patient: This woman had given birth four times. Perhaps they were all girls, or perhaps any sons did not survive. Then there was a ten year period with no more births. Note that the woman is 32 at the time of treatment, meaning that she had four children by the time she was 22.

Chāng 娼, here translated as *female performer*, is often translated as prostitute, but *A Student's Dictionary of Classical and Medieval Chinese*[82] assures us that, at least in ancient times, this was not the definition. The patient's husband spent time with female performers (dancers, singers, etc.). In Chinese singular and plural are not automatically expressed, so it is possible that this was one performer, not many. This contributed to the patient's anger (one cause of her inability to have children) but the presence of a sexually transmitted disease cannot be ruled out.

The Disease: The first paragraph describes a woman with what we call *premenstrual syndrome* today. One can understand why from her circumstances. Rage alterrnated with suppressed emotions and the resulting constraint and fire consumed her right qì.

The woman developed white *lín*-dribbling (*bái lín* 白淋). The term *lín*-dribbling usually denotes various types of difficult urination. Here it seems to refer to a vaginal discharge instead. The next paragraph includes a quotation from *Mài Jué* about white [vaginal] *dài*-discharge that makes this clear. Considering the circumstances, this discharge could be a sexually transmitted disease brought home by the husband.

---

82. By Paul W. Kroll, published by Brill in 2015.

Cited Texts: *Míng Táng Zhēn Jiǔ* 《明堂鍼灸》 (Acupuncture-Moxibustion of the Bright Hall) is an alternate name for *Míng Táng Jīng* 《明堂經》 (Bright Hall Classic), edited during the Western and Eastern *Hàn* dynasties (between 138 B.C.E.-106 C.E.) but this book has since been lost. Much of it was reprinted during the *Sòng* dynasty as Volumes 99 and 100 of *Tài Píng Shèng Huì Fāng* 《太平聖惠方》 (Sage-like Prescriptions of Tài Píng Era). However no statement that "acupuncture cuts off childbearing but three complete applications of moxibustion enables a person to give birth" can be found in it. In the context of Chinese medicine, the term *Míng Táng* 明堂 refers to books, sections of books, or diagrams about acu-moxa points. Tán's statement here does not appear to be a quotation or a paraphrase from a specific book known today. It is a summary of information from different books and from the entries for different points. For example, *Tóng Rén* 《銅人》 (1026, *Sòng*) says acupuncture on Shí Mén (Rèn 5) causes infertility. It also says that three cones of moxibustion on Yīn Lián (LV 11) can cure infertility. Many later books passed on statements such as these.

This is the only case of Tán's that refers to sources other than formula books.

Treatment: Tán applied a lot of moxibustion on the lower abdomen to warm the *dān tián* region and the Chōng and Rén Vessels. This is an effective treatment for a cold and painful lower abdomen.

For *Hé Shǒu Wū Wán*: See Case 20.

It took three more years, but in the end, the woman was able to have a son.

Case 24: Irregular Menstruation

一婦人，年五十三歲，因經事不調，元氣甚弱，得患氣血俱虛之症。某復其脈，心經脈甚浮洪，有六止。其婦多勞碌以致，傷心；心乃一身之主，其心火動，經事不期而行，倍加虛弱。

Because the menstrual period of a 53 year old woman was irregular and her original qì was very weak, she suffered an ailment with deficiency of both qì and blood. I rechecked her pulse; the heart channel pulse was extremely floating and surging, and it would stop for six beats [irregular pulse]. The reason was that the woman was often taxed from toil which damaged the heart. The heart is the master of the whole body; when her heart fire stirred, menstruation did not come when expected, increasing her deficiency and weakness.

某用補虛之劑兼神砂丸，服之畧可不得全除。

I used a prescription to supplement deficiency together with *Shén Shā Wán*. She took it, improving slightly, but it did not completely eliminate her ailment.

某意謂此婦即是血氣不調，後用歸珀丸。又用升提理氣煎藥，服之即愈，其婦精健如舊。

My opinion was that this woman [suffered from] unregulated blood and qì. Then I used *Guī Pò Wán*. In another visit I used a decoction to uplift and rectify qì [modified *Bǔ Zhōng Yì Qì Tāng* and *Èr Chén Tāng*, see below]. She took these formulas and then recovered; the woman became mentally sharp and strong like before.

補中益氣湯兼二陳湯，加：

Bǔ Zhōng Yì Qì Tāng together with *Èr Chén Tāng*, adding:

122

wǔ wèi	五味		30 pcs	
xiāng fù	香附	stir-fry until black	1 qián	3.73 g

又服丸藥歸珀丸（出《摘玄方》）。

In another visit she took the herbal pill *Guī Pò Wán* (from *Zhāi Xuán Fāng*).

dāng guī	當歸		2 liǎng	74.6 g
hǔ pò	琥珀		0.5 qián	1.87 g
xiāng fù	香附	Soak in child's urine (*tóng biàn*) for three days. Divide it into four parts: soak one part in vinegar, soak one part in liquor, soak one part in rice washing water, soak one part in salt water; soak each for three days. Stir-fry.	1 jīn	596.8 g
		add 加		
fú líng	茯苓		2 liǎng	74.6 g
zé lán	澤蘭		2 liǎng	74.6 g

Powder the above and make pills with vinegar and flour-paste; the pills should be the size of *wú zǐ* (about 0.6-0.9 centimeters in diameter). Take them on an empty stomach swallowing them with hot salt water, a hundred pills each dose.

Notes on Case 24

The Disease: At 53, today we would attribute her irregular periods to menopause. Perhaps if her menstrual periods ceased without any other symptoms, it would not be considered pathology. However, this woman was diagnosed with qì deficiency and heart fire. While specific symptoms are not mentioned, the deficiency was probably more obvious since that was the original diagnosis. Tán double-checked and found that the heart pulse was not deficient. This confirmed that the condition was not pure deficiency. The heart fire might may have manifested in insomnia or with emotional outbursts.

Treatment: Tán's first attempt at treatment was mildly successful. She used *Shén Shā Wán*: Tán did not mention the source. It is from Volume 24 of *Jī Fēng Pǔ Jì Fāng*.[83]

神砂丸
Shén Shā Wán (from Volume 24 of *Jī Fēng Pǔ Jì Fāng*)
Shén Shā Pills

chén shā	辰砂	1 liǎng	37.3 g
nì fèn	膩粉	1 liǎng	37.3 g
dìng fèn	定粉	0.5 liǎng	18.65 g
fèn shuāng	粉霜	1.5 qián	5.6 g
bái dìng xiāng	白丁香	half of a *zì* 字.*	
shè xiāng	麝香	a small amount	

Powder the above and make pills the size of mung beans with a grain drink (*Sù Mǐ Yǐn* 粟米飲). Pinch the round pills into flat cakes. Quick-fry them over gentle heat until they turn purple. Each dose is 1 pill after meals, dissolved in a grain drink (*Sù Mǐ Yǐn*).
For accumulations and stagnation in deficiency cases, transforms phlegm drool and milk *pǐ*-aggregations. *Shén Shā Wán* was originally a pediatric formula.

* *Zì* 字 is an ancient measurement. There are four characters (*zì* 字) written on one side of the old coins that have a square hole in the center. One *zì* is as much herbal powder as it takes to cover one of the characters. This is half of that amount. It seems like a minuscule amount in comparison to the other ingredients.

Perhaps the *Shén Shā Wán* resolved the heart fire, because later formulas did not address that. She supplemented, uplifted, and rectified qì with *Bǔ Zhōng Yì Qì Tāng* (see Case 3) together with *Èr Chén Tāng* (see Case 6).

The recipe for *Guī Pò Wán* is given in the case, but it does not seem to be a commonly used formula. It is similar in both preparation and ingredients to *Sì Zhì Xiāng Fù Wán*, which is found in Case 27. It was used to regulate blood and qì.

In the end, the woman became mentally sharp and strong like before.

---

83. *Jī Fēng Pǔ Jì Fāng* 張銳《雞峰普濟方》is attributed to Zhāng Ruì, *Sòng*.

Case 25: Abdominal Lumps

一婦人，年二十四歲，在室富貴兩全，受用甚厚，既嫁翁姑
雖富，嚴謹慳恪，況夫亦年少，不能處事，父母亦遊宦，其
婦憂愁成疾，結塊腹中三年。服藥不愈。某詢其疾久，非專
服藥可能除。某就取灸：

Before a 24 year old woman was married, she received both wealth and honor
and was completely and profoundly comfortable; after being married, her
parents-in-law were strict and miserly even though they were wealthy. Furthermore, her husband was young and unable to deal with affairs.[84] Her parents
were also officials posted far away. Three years ago, the woman's sorrow and
worry developed into the illness of a nodular lump in her abdomen. She had
taken medicine but did not recover. I had inquired into her illness for a long
time [and I realized that] focusing on taking medicine would not eliminate it. I
then selected the following for moxibustion:

Shàng Wǎn (Rèn 13)	上脘	single point
Zhōng Wǎn (Rèn 12)	中脘	single point
Xià Wǎn (Rèn 10)	下脘	single point
Shí Guān (non-channel)	食關	bilateral point

各灸一十四壯。

Fourteen cones of moxibustion were applied on each point.

後服香砂調中湯（出《摘玄》）、枳實丸（出《丹溪方》）
。其塊自消，遂獲全愈。

Afterwards she took *Xiāng Shā Tiáo Zhōng Tāng* (from *Zhāi Xuán*) and *Zhǐ Shí
Wán* (from *Dān Xī Fāng*). The lump dispersed itself, and she then was able to
completely recover.

---

84. This probably meant the husband could or would not protect his wife against his
parents.

Notes on Case 25

The Patient: This woman grew up with a loving family, but suddenly found herself with no support from her husband, her in-laws, or her parents. It must have been a lonely existence. According to Chapter 39 of *Sù Wèn*, emotions make qì move in contrary ways. When qì moves improperly, so does blood. This is how the abdominal lump developed.

Treatment: Tán had been treating this patient with herbal medicine for a while, but the patient did not recover. Because of this, Tán decided to try moxibustion. For discussion of the moxibustion treatment, see Case 10.

At this time, the location and function of the point called Lóng Xìng 隆興 is unknown. This is the only time Tán prescribed it in her published case studies. It is possible that this is the same as Xìng Lóng 興隆 which has the same characters in reverse order. Xìng Lóng is located 1 cùn above the umbilicus and one cùn to each side. Based on the location of at least the first three points, the lump was probably in the upper abdomen and may be related to food and digestion.

The patient took *Xiāng Shā Tiáo Zhōng Tāng* (from *Zhāi Xuán*). *Zhāi Xuán* is no longer extant. There are no results in searches for a formula by this name that pre-dates Tán. However, formulas published in later books may have been around for a long time, but the previous references were lost. This formula may be similar to the one by the same name in Volume 3 of *Shòu Shì Bǎo Yuán*[85] which was published about a hundred years later:

---

85. *Shòu Shì Bǎo Yuán* 《壽世保元 》 was written by Gōng Tíngxián 龔廷賢 (1522 - 1619) and published in 1615.

香砂調中湯
Xiāng Shā Tiáo Zhōng Tāng (from *Shòu Shì Bǎo Yuán*)
Xiāng Shā Decoction to Regulate the Center

huò xiāng	藿香		1.2 qián	4.51 g
shā rén	砂仁		1.2 qián	4.51 g
cāng zhú	蒼朮	dry-fried	1.5 qián	5.6 g
hòu pǔ	厚樸	stir-fried with ginger juice	1 qián	3.73 g
chén pí	陳皮	remove the white part	1 qián	3.73 g
bàn xià	半夏	stir-fried with ginger juice	1 qián	3.73 g
bái fú líng	白茯苓	remove the peel	1 qián	3.73 g
shén qū	神曲	dry-fried	1 qián	3.73 g
zhǐ shí	枳實	dry-fried with wheat bran	1 qián	3.73 g
qīng pí	青皮	remove the pulp	1 qián	3.73 g
shān zhā ròu	山楂肉		1 qián	3.73 g
bái zhú	白朮		1.5 qián	5.6 g
zhì gān cǎo	炙甘草		0.3 qián	1.12g

File one package into powder. Add *shēng jiāng*, boil and take.
For food damage to the spleen and stomach with damp phlegm and qì constraint; food accumulations make distention and fullness of the heart region and abdomen.

If this is the correct formula, it also points toward food and digestion as part of the pattern. If so, beginning treatment with moxibustion is smart, as herbs need to be processed by the spleen and stomach. If they are already ailing, moxibustion may be better received by the body than herbal medicine.

Zhǐ Shí Wán treats various kinds of abdominal lumps:

枳實丸
Zhǐ Shí Wán (from *Dān Xī Xīn Fǎ*)
Zhǐ Shí Pill

bái zhú	白朮	2 liǎng	74.6 g
zhǐ shí	枳實	1 liǎng	37.3 g
bàn xià	半夏	1 liǎng	37.3 g

shén qū	神曲	1 liǎng	37.3 g
mài yá	麥芽	1 liǎng	37.3 g
jiāng huáng	薑黃	0.5 liǎng	18.65 g
chén pí	陳皮	0.5 liǎng	18.65 g
mù xiāng	木香	1.5 qián	5.6 g
shān zhā	山楂	1 liǎng	37.3 g

Powder the above, make into pills the size of *wú tóng zǐ* 梧桐子 (about 0.6-0.9 centimeters in diameter) using rice steamed with *hé yè* 荷葉. Each dose is 100 pills, taken after meals with a decoction of ginger.

Case 26: *Wěi*-Atrophy 2

一婦人，年三十歳，得患氣痿之症。曉夜不睡，半年不能起床；諸藥無效，某復其脈，似勞碌太過，以致虛損。又因受大氣一塲，遂成此疾。某用人參六君子湯。又服瓊玉膏。漸漸安神，得睡。服藥兩月，遂得全愈。

A 30 year old woman suffered the ailment of qì *wěi*-atrophy. She could not sleep in the day or at night, and was unable to get out of bed for half a year. Various medicines had no effect, so I retook her pulse. It seemed that taxation from too much toil resulted in deficiency harm. Also because she endured an episode of great anger, she then developed this illness. I used *Rén Shēn Liù Jūn Zǐ Tāng*. She also took *Qióng Yù Gāo*. Her spirit calmed little by little and she was able to sleep. She took the medicine for two months, and then completely recovered.

人參六君子湯，加：

Rén Shēn Liù Jūn Zǐ Tāng, adding:

fú shén	茯神	2 qián	7.46 g
chái hú	柴胡	1 qián	3.73 g
shēng má	升麻	3 fēn	1.12 g

mù xiāng	木香	2 fēn	0.75 g
yuǎn zhì	遠志	1 qián	3.73 g
shén shā	神砂	5 fēn	1.87 g
huáng lián	黃蓮	1 qián	3.73 g
bàn xià	半夏	1 qián	3.73 g
xiāng fù	香附	1 qián	3.73 g

[Boil in] two cups of water with three slices of ginger. Take between meals.

Notes on Case 26

The Disease: Qì *wěi*-atrophy (氣痿) here indicates *wěi*-atrophy due to qì deficiency. This is usually because of excessive toil or poor diet, which damage the spleen-stomach. As a result, insufficient post-heaven qì is made, and the limbs (which resonate with the spleen-stomach) do not get nourished. In this case, the main symptom supporting a diagnosis of *wěi*-atrophy is that she could not get out of bed for a long time. Anger is mentioned so the spleen-stomach deficiency may be due to liver qì constraint in addition to excessive toil. The heart and spirit also seem to be an important aspect of her problem, yet are not mentioned in the diagnosis. The disquieted spirit can be explained by a lack of nourishment since post-heaven qì and blood are lacking.

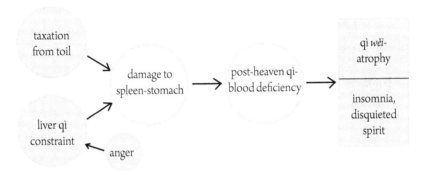

129

Treatment: The treatment was *Liù Jūn Zǐ Tāng* with additions:

六君子湯
Liù Jūn Zǐ Tāng
Six Gentlemen Decoction

rén shēn	人參
bái zhú	白朮
fú líng	茯苓
gān cǎo	甘草
shā rén	砂仁
chén pí	陳皮

Tán's additions

fú shén	茯神
chái hú	柴胡
shēng má	升麻
mù xiāng	木香
yuǎn zhì	遠志
shén shā	神砂
huáng lián	黃蓮
bàn xià	半夏
xiāng fù	香附

Boil in water with three slices of ginger and one piece of *dà zǎo*.

Tán probably substituted *fú shén* for *fú líng*; no need to have both. The added herbs calm the spirit, harmonize the liver and spleen, and raise and regulate qì

For more details on *Rén Shēn Liù Jūn Zǐ Tāng* and for *Qióng Yù Gāo*, see Case 18. The patients in both these cases suffered *wěi*-atrophy.

Case 27: Frequent Miscarriage 2

一婦人，年三十六歲，生四胎後，三胎將三四箇月，即墮。其夫因富貴，深憂無子，甚欲娶妾，其婦與某商議，無計阻，當憂忿太過，家事頗繁，愈加不能成胎。

After giving birth four times, a 36 year old woman miscarried three times when she was three or four months into the pregnancy. Because her husband was wealthy and high ranking, he was profoundly worried about not having a son. He very much wanted to take on a concubine. The woman discussed it with me; she did not have a plan to block it, but enduring the sorrow and anger was too much. Matters of running the household were quite numerous, further adding to her inability to become pregnant.

某意謂勞怒傷情內火便動，亦能墮胎。遂與四製香附丸，又調經益氣湯（俱出《摘玄方》）加

My opinion was that this was taxation and anger; internal fire was stirred up from emotional damage and was then able to cause the miscarriages. I gave her *Sì Zhì Xiāng Fù Wán*. In another visit I gave her *Tiáo Jīng Yì Qì Tāng* (both from *Zhāi Xuán Fāng*), adding:

bái fú líng	白茯苓		1 qián	3.73 g
chuān xiōng	川芎		1 qián	3.73 g
xiāng fù	香附	stir-fry until black	1 qián	3.73 g
huáng qín	黃芩	stir-fried with liquor	1.5 qián	5.6 g

半年後有胎。又服安胎末藥：

A half year later she was pregnant. She also took powdered herbs to calm the fetus:

shǔ wěi huáng qín	鼠尾黃芩	vinegar processed	2 liǎng	74.6 g
bái zhú	白朮		2 liǎng	74.6 g

右為末，每服二錢，紫蘇湯下。次年五月，遂生一子。

Powder the above. Each dose is 2 qián (7.46 grams) swallowed with a decoction of *zǐ sū*. In the fifth month of the next year [around June of the Western calendar], she gave birth to a son.

Notes on Case 27

The Patient: Although not stated, the first four children must have been girls, or if sons were born, they must not have survived.

Treatment: *Sì Zhì Xiāng Fù Wán* as originally from *Hé Shì Jì Shēng Lùn*. Not much is known about this document, although it was cited in other books.

四製香附丸
Sì Zhì Xiāng Fù Wán (from Volume 7 of *Hé Shì Jì Shēng Lùn*)
Xiāng Fù Pill with Four Preparations

xiāng fu	香附	divide into four portions, soak each portion in one of the following: child's urine,* liquor, vinegar, and water from rinsing rice. If it is spring, soak for 3 days, 1 day in summer, and 5 days in winter. Dry in the sun.	1 jīn	586.8 g
dāng guī	當歸	washed in liquor	1 liǎng	37.3 g

Powder the above and make into water pills. Each dose is 3 qián (11.2 grams) taken with clear soup.
Regulates menstruation, nourishes blood, promotes proper flow of qì, and treats infertility.

* Child's urine was commonly used in ancient times, generally from a prepubescent male. It was used in cooking formulas or for processing herbs. It is generally considered to be heat-clearing.

This formula is similar in both preparation and ingredients to *Guī Pò Wán* (lacking only the *hǔ pò*), which is found in Case 24.

Tiáo Jīng Yì Qì Tāng is from *Zhāi Xuán Fāng* (no longer extant). There is a *Tiáo Jīng Yì Qì Wán* (pill, not decoction) from *Huó Rén Fāng*.[86] The formula Tán used may be similar.

調經益氣丸
Tiáo Jīng Yì Qì Wán (from Volume 6 of *Huó Rén Fāng*)
Pill to Regulate Menstruation and Boost Qì

shēng dì	生地	8 liǎng	298.4 g
dāng guī	當歸	5 liǎng	186.5 g
bái sháo	白芍	5 liǎng	186.5 g
zhì xiāng fù	製香附	5 liǎng	186.5 g
dān pí	丹皮	5 liǎng	186.5 g
fú líng	茯苓	3 liǎng	111.9 g
dù zhòng	杜仲	3 liǎng	111.9 g
gǒu qǐ zǐ	枸杞子	3 liǎng	111.9 g
bái zhú	白朮	3 liǎng	111.9 g
niú xī	牛膝	3 liǎng	111.9 g
zé xiè	澤瀉	3 liǎng	111.9 g
chuān xiōng	川芎	2 liǎng	74.6 g
huáng qí	黃耆	2 liǎng	74.6 g
yán hú	延胡	2 liǎng	74.6 g
chén pí	陳皮	2 liǎng	74.6 g

Powder and make into honey pills. Each dose is 3 to 5 qián (11.19 - 18.65 grams) taken with boiled water in the early morning on an empty stomach.

This formula supplements both qì and blood, opens up constraint, normalizes qì flow, enriches yīn, and clears heat. It is indicated for insufficiency of original qì in females with loss of circulation leading to qì stagnation or constraint and pain in the chest or abdomen. Since *yíng* and blood are deficient, the ability to nourish is lost. With blood deficiency comes blood heat so menstruation becomes irregular. The hundred diseases erupt and the shining of body and spirit is decreased.

The unnamed formula of *huáng qín* and *bái zhú* was seen in a previous case. See Case 4 for discussion of this formula and the mechanisms of miscarriage.

---

86. Not much is known about *Huó Rén Fāng* 《活人方》. It is also called *Huó Rén Fāng Huì Biān* 《活人方汇编》.

Case 28: Severe Food Accumulation 1

一女子，方年六歲，父母愛甚不惜飲食。元宵恣意多食糖圓
子，約及兩箇月將死。諸藥不效，無計可治。某將追積丸（
出《摘玄方》）。漸漸捱下，圓子數十枚，白幕包裹，仍不
曾消，不久其患即愈。

The parents of a girl who had just turned six loved her a lot and were not stingy with drink and food. On the night of the Lantern Festival, the girl did as she pleased and ate too much *táng yuán zǐ* (a special sweet served at this time). After about two months, she was close to death. Various medicines were ineffective and [other doctors] had no plan for treating it. I used *Zhuī Jī Wán* (Pill to Chase Accumulations) (from *Zhāi Xuán Fāng*). One at a time several tens of *yuán zǐ* came out in the stool, wrapped up in white 'veils,' still undigested. Before long her suffering recovered.

Notes on Case 28

General Background: The Lantern Festival (*yuán xiāo jié* 元宵節) falls on the fifteenth day of the first lunar month (*yuán xiāo* - the full moon in the first lunar month). It is the last day of New Year celebrations. People decorate their houses with special lanterns and carry them in the streets. A special sweet is eaten on this day, called *táng yuán zǐ* or *yuán xiāo* 元宵. It is made from glutinous rice flour and filled with a paste of red beans, peanuts, or black sesame seeds.

The Disease: The girl ate too many *táng yuán zǐ*. The glutinous rice stuck in her digestive tract and she could no longer eat.

Treatment: *Zhuī Jī Wán* was prescribed in this and the next case. Its stated source, *Zhāi Xuán Fāng*, is no longer extant. There is a formula in *Lǔ Fǔ Jìn Fāng*[87] with a similar name: *Zhuī Chóng Qǔ Jī Wán*. Even though this book was published later, it is probably similar to the formula Tán used.

87. *Lǔ Fǔ Jìn Fāng*《魯府禁方》was written by Gōng Tíngxián 龔廷賢 (1522 - 1619).

追蟲取積丸
Zhuī Chóng Qǔ Jī Wán (from Volume 2 of *Lǔ Fǔ Jīn Fāng*)
Pill to Chase out Worms and Aim at Accumulations

hēi qiān niú	黑牽牛	powdered	4 liǎng	149.2 g
bīng láng	檳榔	powdered	4 liǎng	149.2 g
bā dòu	巴豆	remove the shell	2 liǎng	74.6 g
dà zào jiǎo	大皂角	a half cùn length		20 pcs

Put the *bā dòu* and *zào jiǎo* into a pot with 3 bowls of water, boil it down to 1 bowl, and remove the dregs. Mix the liquid with the other two powdered herbs and make it into pills the size of *wú tóng zǐ* 梧桐子 (about 0.6-0.9 centimeters in diameter). Dry them in the sun. Sprinkle a bowl of water on them and dry them in the sun again; do this two times (for a total of three dryings). After this, they will be shiny like crystals. Each dose is 3 qián (11.2 grams). During the fourth watch (1-3 a.m.), mix it with granulated sugar (*shā tang* 砂糖) and swallow it. If the accumulation does not move, drink a mouthful of hot water to hasten it; it will move 11-12 times (meaning bowel movements). Afterwards, it is good to be on a restricted diet for five to seven days.

This formula can aim at worms if someone has worms; it can aim at accumulations if someone has accumulations.

In this and the next case, the problem is food accumulations, not worms, but this formula treats either by violently expelling whatever is in the digestive tract.

Case 29: Severe Food Accumulation 2

一婦人，年二十八歲，造酒為生，終日忙甚，失落銀挑心一箇，一日夜無獲，湯水不進，況有胎五箇月。其姑憐其為財痛傷受餓煨米餅二枚，食之一枚，停於中脘，一月餘不進米粒，將欲命絕，遂置衾棺。其姑問某，含悲泣訴，得患之情。

A 28 year old woman brewed liquor to make a living and was extremely busy all day long. She lost a silver hair ornament[88] and spent one day and night

---

88. The meaning of *tiāo xīn* 挑心 is not totally certain. It seems to be some kind of ornamental hairpin. Whatever it was, it was an object of value to the patient.

searching but could not find it. She did not eat anything and moreover she was five months pregnant. Her aunt [father's sister] pitied her because she was so distressed over something of material value and suffered from hunger, so she gave the woman two baked rice cakes. The woman ate one, but it got stuck at Zhōng Wǎn [the middle of the stomach, the region of Rèn 12]. For more than a month she could not even swallow a grain of rice and was about to die. They set up her burial clothes and coffin. Full of grief and sobbing her sorrows, the aunt asked me how she got into this situation.

某將追積丸方（ 見前 ），磨辟灌之，少停追下其積，青黯色，米餅未消 。患者甦醒，就吃茶湯 。又與安胎順氣之劑，調理遂獲痊，安後生一女 。

I used the *Zhuī Jī Wán* formula (see above); I ground it up, opened her mouth, and poured it in. We waited a little while and it pursued the accumulation downward. Green and dark in color, the rice cake had never been digested. The patient revived, woke up, and then drank some tea. I also gave her a prescription to calm the fetus and help qì to flow properly. She took care of herself and was then able to recover. After she returned to health, she gave birth to a girl.

Notes on Case 29

The Disease: This woman was emotionally upset about losing something. She was pregnant and hungry. When she finally ate, the food stuck in her middle *jiāo*. The undigested mass blocked her ability to eat anything else and so she almost died.

Treatment: For *Zhuī Jī Wán*, see the previous case. Since this formula violently expels accumulations from the digestive tract, it is risky for a weak patient and for the pregnancy. But more mild treatments would not be strong enough. Tán took a risk, trying to save the woman's life. The rice cake came out with the stool, undigested but changed to dark green. The risk payed off and both mother and child lived.

In this case, we can surmise that Tán traveled to the patient's dwelling as the patient was semiconscious or unconscious.

Case 30: Tortoise Lump

一婦人，四十九歲，腹中生一龜塊，在左邊，二十七年，如塊轉動，疼至將死，諸藥無効。某與灸：

A 49 year old woman had a tortoise lump growing on the left side of her abdomen for 27 years. If the lump moved, it was painful as if she were about to die. Various medicines lacked results. I gave her moxibustion on:

Zhōng Wǎn (Rèn 12)	中脘	single point
Jiàn Lǐ (Rèn 11)	建里	single point*
Chéng Mǎn (ST 20)	承滿	bilateral point

* Jiàn Lǐ (Rèn 11) is a single point but the original text said "bilateral point." It has been corrected here.

後服蚶殼丸一升（ 出《 摘玄方 》 ）。至今一十餘年，不發其塊，並不轉動 。

Afterwards she took one *shēng* of *Hān Ké Wán* (from *Zhāi Xuán Fāng*). Until now, more than ten years later, the lump has not expanded and has not moved.

Notes on Case 30

The Disease: A tortoise lump would be one shaped like a tortoise shell - oval and hard. The mention of the lump moving is curious. Perhaps it was in the vicinity of the intestines. As stool passed through, it might jostle the lump, causing pain. On the other hand, perhaps the lump was a bolus of parasites that moved on its own. However, the text does not mention any symptoms of parasites and after 27 years, that diagnosis should be obvious.

Treatment: Since herbs had not worked in the past, Tán tried moxibustion instead. Chéng Mǎn (ST 20) is five cùn above the umbilicus and two cùn lateral to the midline. Jiàn Lǐ (Rèn 11) and Zhōng Wǎn (Rèn 12) are on the midline, three and four cùn above the umbilicus respectively. These points were probably in the vicinity of the lump. All these points treat conditions such as abdominal distention and pain.

Hān Ké Wán was originally from Volume 41 of *Jì Yáng Gāng Mù.*[89] The formula consists only of *hān ké* (also called *wǎ lǒng zǐ* 瓦壟子). This shell is calcined with vinegar, crushed 3 times, and powdered. Then it is made into pills with vinegar and flour paste and swallowed with a decoction of ginger. *Hān Ké Wán* treats all types of lumps, concretions, and conglomerations due to qì, blood, or phlegm. Tán did not mention any modifications.

The treatment did not cure the lump, but it did not grow any more and since it did not move, the patient no longer experienced pain.

Case 31: Botched Abortion

一婦人，年三十八歲，曾產十胎後，有孕怕生，因服藥墮胎，不期惡露去多將死，藥三月止存殘命，其母九月間去看，將豬腤肺及風菱與食，自此病加，至次年三月，一向諸食不進，略飲米湯，況經事不行，幾欲命絕。其母特訴此情。某與調理煎藥二帖，二陳湯、四物湯，加：

After a 38 year old woman had already given birth ten times, she was pregnant. The woman feared giving birth again so she took medicine to induce an abortion. She didn't expect so much lochia [literally evil dew] to be discharged and she was on the verge of death. She took medicine for three months, just barely preserving her remaining life. Her mother came to tend to her during the ninth month [around October in the Western calendar]. She brought pork

---

89. *Jì Yáng Gāng Mù* 《濟陽綱目》 (108 volumes) was written by Wǔ Zhīwàng 武之望, and published in 1626 (*Míng*). This was after Tán's book was published, so there must be an earlier, lost source. It is also possible that Tán used a different formula with the same name.

belly and lungs as well as caltrops[90] for the daughter to eat. From that point, the disease increased until the third month of the next year when she was unable to swallow any food and could only drink a little thin rice gruel. Furthermore her menstrual period did not come. She almost died. Her mother explained the situation to me. I gave her two packets of a decoction to help her recover, *Èr Chén Tāng* and *Sì Wù Tāng*, adding:

shā rén	砂仁	1 qián	3.73 g
shén qū	神麴	1 qián	3.73 g
xiāng fù	香附	1 qián	3.73 g
zhǐ shí	枳實	1 qián	3.73 g

並阿魏丸（出《摘玄方》）。其母將藥回歸，舉家哀哭。先以煎藥一盞，撬開患人口，灌之，當得甦醒。又服煎藥二十帖，丸藥一升，遂得全俞。

At the same time I gave her *Ā Wèi Wán* (from *Zhāi Xuán Fāng*). Her mother took the herbs with her and returned, finding the whole family weeping in sorrow. They first used a cup of the decocted herbs, forcing the patient's mouth open and pouring it in. Right then she revived and woke up. She additionally took twenty packets of the decocted medicine and one *shēng* (1073.7 grams) of the herbal pills, and then completely recovered.

Notes on Case 31

The Patient: Why did the woman try to induce an abortion? Perhaps she was poor and ten children are already quite a few. Perhaps she was exhausted from all those pregnancies, aging, and whatever work she needed to do. Perhaps in the past childbirth was difficult or had complications. There are many possibilities but we do not know the reason.

The Disease: We also do not know in which month she terminated the pregnancy. In any case, afterwards the patient had a discharge that did not stop and weakened her tremendously. Tán implied that the food the

---

90. Caltrops are large starchy seeds similar to water chestnuts.

mother brought was inappropriate. The woman became progressively weaker, in part from her condition and in part because she could not eat.

General Background: This is a case where Tán did not actually see the patient. Travelling was not easy for an upper class woman at the time unless she had a male relative to escort her. Apparently she could not go in this case, so Tán gave the herbs (or perhaps a prescription for the herbs) to the mother. Lower class women were somewhat freer to move around outside the home as they often needed to for work. The patient's mother must have been lower class or her desperation pushed her to go out.

This is the only case of Tán's that is clearly a long distance consultation. Other (male) doctors of the time also prescribed herbs based on letters from patients or descriptions from relatives of the patient. Wāng Jī was an example of this. In his case study collection, called *Shí Shān Yī Àn* (Medical Cases of Stone Mountain),[91] Wāng documented a number of long distance consultations.

Treatment: For both *Èr Chén Tāng* and *Sì Wù Tāng*, see Case 6.

四物湯
Sì Wù Tāng
Decoction of Four Substances

dāng guī	當歸	
chuān xiōng	川芎	
bái sháo	白芍	
shú dì huáng	熟地黃	

二陳湯
Èr Chén Tāng
Decoction of Two Aged Ingredients

bàn xià	半夏	
jú hóng	橘紅	
fú líng	茯苓	

---

91. 汪機《石山醫案》 c. 1531 (*Míng*), published twenty years after Tán's book.

gān cǎo	甘草

usually cooked with ginger 薑 and wū méi 烏梅.

Tán's additions

shā rén	砂仁
shén qū	神麴
xiāng fù	香附
zhǐ shí	枳實

This combination would nourish and move blood, regulate qì, and transform phlegm and dampness.

Here is *Ā Wèi Wán* from *Dān Xī Xīn Fǎ*:

阿魏丸
Ā Wèi Wán (from *Dān Xī Xīn Fǎ*)
Ā Wèi Pill

shān zhā	山楂		3 liǎng	111.9 g
shí jiǎn	石鹼		1 qián	11.2 g
bàn xià	半夏	soaked in zào jiǎo 皂角 water until it fully penetrates, dried in the sun	1 liǎng	37.3 g

Powder the above with 0.5 liǎng (18.65 grams) of ā wèi. Make into pills with a vinegar and flour paste. Each dose is 30 pills, swallowed with clear broth.

Treats food accumulations, meat accumulations, pediatric food accumulations, a spider-like abdomen (big belly but small limbs), abdominal pain, white turbid urine, pediatric abdominal distention, and phlegm-rheum that becomes an accumulation.

Apparently Tán felt that the most urgent problem was food accumulation blocking the digestive tract since the disease worsened after the mother brought pork and caltrops. There was no chance for recovery if the woman could not start eating again. These herbs are milder than *Zhuī Jī Wán* which was used in Cases 28 and 29. In those cases, the patients were younger, had not given birth to ten children, and had not recently suffered losses like this patient after her abortion.

Reading Miscellaneous Records of a Female Doctor

余聞醫家之說有曰：寧醫十男子，不醫一婦人。其所以苦於
醫婦人者，非徒內外相隔，亦由性氣不同之故也。惟婦人醫
婦人，則以己之性氣，度人之性氣；猶兵家所謂以夷攻夷，
而無不克者矣。

I have heard the talk of doctors; they say, "I prefer treating ten men to treating one woman." The reason for their feeling of hardship in treating women is not only due to the separation of inside and outside,[92] it is also because of differences in their temperament. But when a female treats a female, she can estimate the patient's temperament because hers is the same. This is like the military strategy of 'anything can be overcome when one uses barbarians to attack barbarians.'

余內之表姊曰楊孺人談氏，聰明讀書，深達於醫，經驗既
多，爰著《女醫雜言》一書。蓋將大濟乎眾，非止仁其一鄉
一邑而已。

My wife's cousin is Lady Tán;[93] she is intelligent, quite literate, deeply informed in medicine, and already has a lot of experience. Therefore she wrote this book *Miscellaneous Records of a Female Doctor*. It will probably be a great assistance to a multitude of people; it will not just provide compassion for one village or one city.[94]

若孺人者，奚復有前所言之苦哉，然則是編之作較之班姬之
賦，衛夫人之書，與朱淑真之詩；其用心得失，豈不大有可
議者耶。

---

92. 'Inside' refers to the domain of women; the 'outside' world was the domain of men. There were different standards of behavior governing each and it was awkward for unrelated males and females to interact. The next part of this sentence implies that it is not only a question of etiquette, but since the nature or temperament of the sexes was seen as being different, male doctors could not really understand female patients.
93. The exact cousin relationship is unknown.
94. By treating patients, Tán benefits those who are near, but by writing a book, many more people may benefit from her insights.

Lady Tán has also suffered like her predecessors; this composition can be compared to the odes of Bān Jī,[95] the calligraphy of Lady Wèi,[96] or with the poetry of Zhū Shūzhēn.[97] There will be a lot of different opinions regarding the merits and faults of her motivation [for writing this book]!

鄉進士仝邑朱恩題

Provincial Graduate from the same city [as Tán], Zhū Ēn inscribed this [undated]

---

95. Bān Jī 班姬 (circa 45-117, *Hàn*): A female historian and author who wrote *Dōng Zhēng Fù*《東征賦》(Odes of a Journey East) and *Nǚ Jiè*《女誡》(Lessons for Women), as well as finishing her brother Bān Gù's 班固 book *Hàn Shū*《漢書》 (Book of Hàn History) after he died. Bān Jī and the next two famous women mentioned by the author of this postscript made extraordinary achievements. In this way, Tán Yǔnxián is like them, according to Zhū Ēn.
96. Lady Wèi 衛夫人 refers to Wèi Shuò 衛鑠 (272-349, *Jìn* dynasty). She was a famous calligrapher.
97. Zhū Shūzhēn 朱淑真 (1135-1180, Southern *Sòng*) was a female poet.

Postscript to the Second Edition of Miscellaneous Records of a Female Doctor

祖姑楊孺人，以女醫名邑中，壽終九十有六。生平活人不可
以數計。余在韶齔，目覩其療婦人病，應手如脫，不稱女中
盧扁哉？

My paternal grand-aunt, Lady Tán Yǔnxián, was a female doctor who was
famous in her town. She died of old age at 96. Over the course of her life, the
people she saved cannot be counted. When I was losing my milk teeth, I saw
her treating women with my own eyes; their diseases responded to her hand as
if she simply cast them off. Can we not call her the female Biǎn Què?[98]

第余聞活人眾者其後必昌，孺人之子濂既早亡；孫喬復以株
連蔽罪死，爰室祀遂斬焉。豈余聞諸史冊者，不足憑乎？為
之搤腕者久矣。

I have heard that the descendants of someone who saves a large group of
people will prosper, but Lady Tán's son [Yáng] Lián died early; then her grandson [Yáng] Qiáo was implicated in a criminal case; he was sentenced to death,
his descendants were killed, and he was beheaded.[99] How could what I heard
from the historical records be so unreliable? This upset me for a long time and I
couldn't let go of it.

邇閒居多暇檢先世遺澤，得余大父大邑府君手書有《女醫雜
言》跋語。余竊謂得是編行世，則孺人之名將藉是不朽。多
方搆之弗得。有客郭寒江氏，持是編授余曰：聞足下將先人
之業是修，請以是書備記室之錄。余再拜受命。

98. Biǎn Què 扁鵲 was an early legendary doctor said to have the skills to raise the
dead.
99. It is likely that the 'crime' was political in nature; if it had been a theft or murderer,
only the criminal himself would be punished. Destroying the whole family implies
a political crime. Since Tán lived to be 96 years old, she surely was alive when her
son died since it is said that he died early. We do not know the year her grandson was
executed, but it is quite possible that Tán was alive then too. Having no male heir was
considered to be tragic as there was no one to make offerings to the ancestors and no
one to carry on the family name.

Recently, when I was not busy and had spare time at home, I examined the things left behind by my ancestors. I found my late grandfather's handwritten Postscript to *Miscellaneous Records of a Female Doctor*.[100] I really wanted to get the book so it could be known again and Lady Tán's fame would have the chance to become immortal. I tried everything possible to find it, but I could not. Then a visitor, Mr. Guō Hánjiāng, came holding this piece of writing. He gave it to me saying, "I heard you want to revise this undertaking of your ancestor; please receive this book and make a copy of it in your study." I bowed twice and accepted his offer.

展卷莊讀，皆正德庚午前所識，庚午後年益高，術益神，廼
無復識而傳之也者，其信然乎；抑嘗識之而今已覆瓿耶。

I spread out the volume to give it a serious reading; all [the cases] were recorded before the *gēng wǔ* year of Zhèngdé's reign (1510).[101] As [Tán] grew older during the years after *gēng wǔ* (1510), her skills became even more magical. Is it possible that she did not continue recording [her cases] to pass them on? Or perhaps she recorded them but now they have already been used to cover sauce jars [they were considered worthless and were lost].

矧是編先嘗鑴諸方板，里中先達邵文莊公暨茹少㝯公輩，素
重名義不侵，為許可題跋中所稱述源流治驗若指掌，良足為
孺人重矣。今此板無有存焉者，傷哉。

Besides this, [there was the issue of the whereabouts of] all the original printing plates engraved for this book. Mister Shào Wénzhuāng and Mister Rú Shǎocān[102] were well-known elders from her village who always valued their reputations and would not do anything to damage it; they agreed to write prefaces or postscripts in which they very clearly recounted the origin and development of her treatment experience. This was quite valuable for Lady Tán. I was distressed to find that now these plates no longer exist.

---

100. This is the next and final Postscript.
101. 1510 was the year the original edition of *Miscellaneous Words from a Female Doctor* was completed.
102. There are no details available of who these men were, but they must have been eminent in the community at the time. Apparently Mister Shào had an impeccable reputation and had written a preface or postscript for the original book, but it was lost.

斬其祀以故其澤易湮也 。余重濡翰而鐫勒之，則孺人之所為
活人者，不得食報於子孫，尚垂名於世世為不朽哉 。

Tán is cut off from her descendants so it is easy for her good works to fall into oblivion.[103] I moistened my brush to re-copy the book and had the plates engraved. Even though her son and grandson cannot pay back what Lady Tán did to save people, she will still leave a noble name that will not decline in future generations.

萬曆乙酉季春修禊日，姪孫脩百拜敬跋

In the last month of spring in the *yǐ yǒu* year of the reign of Wànlì (1585), on a purification ceremony day, her brother's grandchild [Tán] Xiū respectfully offers this postscript with one hundred obeisances

---

103. Since Tán's direct decendants were dead, there was no one left to promote her memory or to make offerings for her. Her grand-nephew Tán Xiū, the author of this Postcript, wanted to correct this lack by republishing her book.

Postscript to Miscellaneous Records of a Female Doctor

《雜言》若干，則皆吾姊楊孺人所經驗者也。孺人聰慧警
敏，迥出吾兄弟輩，為祖母茹太宜人所鍾愛，飲食動息必
俱。所言莫非醫藥，孺人能入耳即不忘。

All of *Miscellaneous Records* is the experience of my elder sister Lady Yáng [Tán
Yǔnxián]. Lady Tán is intelligent, alert, and perceptive, far beyond anyone in
my brothers' generation [including cousins]. She was cherished by Grandmother Rú; they were always together whether drinking or eating, during
activity or rest. All they talked about was medicine and herbs and anything that
entered Lady Tán's ear was never forgotten.

書得肯綮，長復究極諸家秘要，而通融用之，故在在獲奇
效。鄉鄰女流得疾者，以必延致為喜。晚恐其淪胥而泯乃著
是書。

Her book has captured the critical points through long, repeated, and thorough
research into the secrets of all the schools [of medicine]; it is applied flexibly so
she achieves uncanny efficacy in every case. Ladies of her hometown who were
ill were happy to invite her [to treat them]. She feared that later [these cases]
would all sink into oblivion and be lost, so she wrote this book.

於戲，良醫之功與良相等，右有是言以活人之難也。泝而上
之稱良相者，代不數；稱良醫者，能幾何哉，而況於後世
乎，況於婦人乎。

Sigh! The contributions of a good doctor and a good minister are equivalent.[104]
The words above [in Tán's case studies] can be used to rescue people from their
difficulties. From former times until now, not many people can be counted as
good ministers; how few can be called good doctors! And furthermore in later
times! And even further as a woman!

---

104. This sentence is based on an ancient story. A Northern *Sòng* government official
named Fàn Zhòngyān 范仲淹 (989-1052) is credited with saying, "If I cannot be a
good minister, I will be a good doctor. 不為良相，便為良醫。"

是書之出必有識者，顧余蕪陋罔測微奧，且言不足以信傳，
要不能輕而重之也，雖然，可得軒而輕之耶？敢贅此以俟。

When this book is published, there must be those who see its value; but foolish me, I cannot fathom its profound mysteries so my words are insufficient to convince those who receive it in the future;[105] my praise will not be able to make later people value it; although can one criticize and make light of it? I dare to append this [postscript] and wait [for later people to find value in this book].

正德辛未四月朔旦，京闈壬子舉人，劣弟一鳳拜書

At dawn on the new moon day of the fourth month of the *xīn wèi* year in the reign of Zhèngdé (1511), successful candidate in the examinations at the capital in the *rén zi* year (1492), respectfully written by me, her younger brother [Tán] Yìfèng

---

105. In part, Tán's brother is being modest, but since he is not a doctor, he is also unable to understand the details of the text.

Books Mentioned by Tán in *Miscellaneous Records of a Female Doctor* or in the Prefaces and Postscripts

Zhāi Xuán Fāng 《 摘玄方 》   *Yuán* (元)

    Selected Profound Formulas   Number of Formulas: 14

Full Title: *Dān Xī Zhāi Xuán Fāng* 《 丹溪摘玄方 》

    Selected Profound Formulas from Zhū Dānxī

        Author unkown

                This book is lost.

Dān Xī Fāng 《 丹溪方 》   *Yuán* (元) 1281-1358

    Zhū Dānxī's Formulas   Number of Formulas: 2

      By Zhū Dānxī 朱丹溪

        Probably refers to the collected formulas of Zhū Dānxī, not a particular book.

Shì Xiào Fāng 《 試效方 》 or 《 試効方 》   *Yuán* (元)

    Tested and Effective Formulas   Number of Formulas: 8

Dōng Yuán Shì Xiào Fāng 《 東垣試效方 》

    Tested and Effective Formulas of Lǐ Dōngyuán

      By Luó Qiānfù 羅謙甫

        Luó was a disciple of Lǐ Dōngyuán 李東垣.

Xiù Zhēn Fāng 《 袖珍方 》   *Míng* (明) 1391

    Pocket-Size Formulary   Number of Formulas: 3

      Lǐ Héng et al.李恒

Xiù Zhēn Fāng Dà Quán 《 袖珍方大全 》

    Pocket-Size Formula Collection

        A compilation of useful formulas from other books. This book still exists but is generally unavailable.

Jú Fāng 《 局方 》   *Sòng* (宋) 1078-1085

    Imperial Pharmacy   Number of Formulas: 5

      Compiled by the *Sòng* Imperial Medical Bureau 宋太醫局編

Tài Píng Huì Mín Hé Jì Jú Fāng 《 太平惠民和劑局方 》

    Beneficial Formulas from the Taiping Imperial Pharmacy

        The official *Sòng* dynasty government-published formulary.

Bá Cuì Fāng 《 拔粹方 》   *Yuán* (元) 1308

     Formulas of Outstanding Works   Number of Formulas: 2

         Edited by Dù Sījìng 杜思敬

Jì Shēng Bá Cuì 《 濟生拔粹 》

     Life-Succoring Collection of Outstanding Works

         This book exists but is not available. It is a collection of important works, mainly of Liú Wánsù 劉完素 and his disciples, including Lǐ Dōngyuán 李東垣.

Liáng Fāng 《 良方 》   *Sòng* (宋) 1237

     Good Formulas   Number of Formulas: 1

         By Chén Zìmíng 陳自明

Fù Rén Dà Quán Liáng Fāng 《 婦人大全良方 》

     A Collection of Good Formulas for Women

Also known as *Dà Quán Liáng Fāng* 《 大全良方 》

     A Collection of Good Formulas

         An early book on female specialty.

Shí Xiān Shēng Fāng 《 時先生方 》   Unknown

     Master Shí's Formulas   Number of Formulas: 1

         Unknown

Mài Jué 《 脈訣 》   *Sòng* (宋)

     Rhymed Songs of Pulse   Mentioned once in the cases and once in the Preface.

         By Cuī Jiāyán 崔嘉言

           A pulse poem.

Míng Táng Zhēn Jiǔ 《 明堂鍼灸 》

     Acupuncture-Moxibustion of the Bright Hall   Mentioned once in the cases.

         Here it seems to be a general reference to acupuncture books.

Nán Jīng 《 難經 》   late *Hàn* (漢)

     Classic of Difficult Issues   Mentioned in the Preface.

         Unknown author.

Nèi Zé 《 内則 》   Warring States (戰國)

     Inner Regulations   Mentioned in the Preface.

         Unknown author.

         A section of *Lǐ Jì* 《 禮記 》 (Book of Rites) that discusses the gender role of women.

Books Mentioned in the Translator's Comments or Footnotes

Dān Xī Zhì Fǎ Xīn Yào《丹溪治法心要》   *Yuán* (元) 1281-1358
     The Heart and Essence of Zhū Dānxī's Treatment Methods
         By Zhū Dānxī 朱丹溪

Dān Xī Xīn Fǎ《丹溪心法》   *Yuán* (元) 1281-1358
     Zhū Dānxī's Heart Method
         By Zhū Dānxī 朱丹溪

Dān Xī Xīn Fǎ Fù Yú《丹溪心法附餘》   *Míng* (明) 1536
     An Appendix to Zhū Dānxī's Heart Method
         By Fāng Guǎng 方廣

Běn Cǎo Yǎn Yì Bǔ Yí《本草衍義補遺》   *Yuán* (元) 1281-1358
     Addendum to the Augmented Materia Medica   The *Běn Cǎo Yǎn Yì* was writ-
         By Zhū Dānxī 朱丹溪   ten by Kòu Zōngshì 寇宗奭
                                               in 1116, Northern *Sòng*.

Nèi Wài Shāng Biàn《內外傷辨》   *Jīn* (金) 1231
     Differentiation of Internal and External Damage
         By Lǐ Dōngyuán 李東垣

Lán Shì Mì Cáng《蘭室秘藏》   *Jīn* (金)
     Secrets Hidden in the Orchid Chamber
         By Lǐ Dōngyuán 李東垣

Pí Wèi Lùn《脾胃論》   *Jīn* (金)
     Discussion of the Spleen and Stomach
         By Lǐ Dōngyuán 李東垣

Huáng Dì Sù Wèn Xuān Míng Lùn Fāng《黃帝素問宣明論   *Jīn* (金) 1172
方》
     Elucidated Prescriptions and Expositions of Huángdì's Plain Questions
         By Liú Wánsù 劉完素

Wèi Shēng Bǎo Jiàn《衛生寶鑑》   *Yuán* (元) 1343
     Precious Mirror of Health
         By Luó Tiānyì 羅天益

Zhèng Yīn Mài Zhì《症因脈治》   *Míng*(明)

Disease Cause, Pulse, and Treatment   Revised in *Qīng* by Qín
Huángshì 秦皇士.

By Qín Jīngmíng 秦景明

Chuāng Yáng Jīng Yàn Quán Shū《瘡瘍經驗全書》 *Míng*(明) 1569

Comprehensive Clinical Experience with Skin Diseases On external medicine
(*wài kē*), attributed to Dòu
By Dòu Mènglín 竇夢麟   Hànqīng 竇漢卿 of the *Sòng*
dynasty.

Pǔ Jì Fāng《普濟方》   *Míng*(明) 1406

Formulas for Universal Relief

Sponsored by the *Míng* government.

Yī Jīng Xiǎo Xué《醫經小學》   *Míng*(明) 1388

Primary Studies of the Medical Classics

By Liú Chún 劉純

Jì Shēng Fāng《濟生方》   *Sòng*(宋) 1253

Formulas to Aid Life   Also known as *Yán Shì Jì Shēng
Fāng*《嚴氏濟生方》
By Yán Yònghé 嚴用和   (Master Yán's Formulas to
Aid Life).

Duō Néng Bǐ Shì《多能鄙事》   *Míng*(明) 1311-1375

Many Abilities for Humble Matters

By Liú Jī 劉基

Tàipíng Shèng Huì Fāng《太平圣惠方》 *Sòng*(宋) 992

Sage-like Prescriptions of Tài Píng Era

Edited by Wáng Huáiyǐn et al. 王怀隐

Běn Cǎo Gāng Mù《本草綱目》   *Míng*(明) 1597

The Great Pharmacopeia

By Lǐ Shízhēn 李時珍

Gǔ Jīn Yī Jiàn《古今醫鑑》   *Míng*(明)

Ancient and Modern View of Medicine

By Gōng Xìn 龔信

Shèng Jì Zǒng Lù《聖濟總錄》   *Sòng*(宋) 1117

Complete Record of Sagely Aid

Published by the *Sòng* government.

Hé Shì Jì Shēng Lùn《何氏濟生論》 — Unknown

Mister Hé's Formulas to Aid Life

Author unknown.

Not much is known about this book, although it was cited by other books.

Hóng Shì Jí Yàn Fāng《洪氏集驗方》 — *Sòng* (宋) 1170

Mister Hóng's Collection of Proven Formulas

By Hóng Zūn 洪遵

Jīn Guì Yào Lüè《金匱要略》 — *Hàn* (漢)

Outline of the Golden Cabinet

By Zhāng Zhòngjǐng 張仲景

Shòu Shì Bǎo Yuán《壽世保元》 — *Míng* (明) 1615

Protecting the Origin for Longevity

By Gōng Tíngxián 龔廷賢

Lǔ Fǔ Jìn Fāng《魯府禁方》 — *Míng* (明) 1522-1619

Secret Formulas of Lǔ Fǔ

By Gōng Tíngxián 龔廷賢

Jī Fēng Pǔ Jì Fāng《雞峰普濟方》 — *Sòng* (宋)

Jī Fēng's Formulas for Universal Aid

Attributed to Zhāng Ruì 張銳

Huó Rén Fāng《活人方》 — Unknown

Formulas for the Living

Author unknown.

Also called *Huó Rén Fāng Huì Biān*《活人方汇编》 (Collection of Formulas for the Living). Not much is known this book.

Shí Shān Yī Àn《石山醫案》 — *Míng* (明) 1531

Medical Cases of Stone Mountain

By Wāng Jī 汪機

A record of many of Wāng Jī's cases.

Zhōng Zàng Jīng《中藏經》 — *Sān Guó* (三國) Three Kingdoms

Classic of the Central Viscera

Attributed to Huá Tuó 華佗

It was surely written later, but the time it was written is unknown.

Jiā Yòu Bǔ Zhù Shén Nóng Běn Cǎo《嘉祐補註神農本草》 — *Sòng* (宋) 1060

Jiā Yòu Reign Supplementary Notes on *Shén Nóng Běn Cǎo*.

Published by the *Sòng* government.

Quoted in *Běn Cǎo Gāng Mù* (published in 1597, *Míng*).

Jì Yáng Gāng Mù《濟陽綱目》   *Míng*（明）1626

    Outline of Aiding Yáng

       By Wǔ Zhīwàng 武之望

Tóng Rén《銅人》   *Sòng*（宋）1026

    The Bronze Man   Full Name: *Tóng Rén Shù*

       By Wáng Wéiyī 王惟一   *Xué Zhēn Jiǔ Tú Jīng*《銅人
    腧穴針灸圖經》（The
    Acupuncture-Moxibustion
    Diagram Classic of Points on
    the Bronze Man)

Míng Táng Jīng《明堂經》   *Hàn*（漢）

    Bright Hall Classic   A points book. The original

       Unknown author.   has been lost but much of it
    was copied into later books.

Jiù Táng Shū《舊唐書》   Compiled in the Five Dynas-
    ties and Ten Kingdoms
    Period.

    Old Táng History   A history book.

       Government commissioned.

Sòng Shǐ《宋史》   Compiled during the *Yuán*（
    元）dynasty.

    Sòng History   A history book.

       Government sponsored.

Dōng Zhēng Fù《東征賦》   *Hàn*（漢）45-117

    Odes of a Journey East   Bān Jī was a female historian
    and author.

       By Bān Jī 班姬

Nǚ Jiè《女誡》   *Hàn*（漢）45-117

    Lessons for Women   Bān Jī was a female historian
    and author.

       By Bān Jī 班姬

Hàn Shū《漢書》   *Hàn*（漢）

    Book of Hàn History   This book was completed by

       By Bān Gù 班固   his sister Bān Jī after Bān Gù
    died.

Translator's Bibliography

Directly mentioning Tán or regarding women and medicine in China

Furth, Charlotte, *A Flourishing Yin: Gender in China's Medical History: 960-1665*; University of California Press (1999).

Tán, Yǔnxián, *Miscellaneous Records of a Female Doctor (nǚ yī zá yán)*; Ancient Chinese Medicine Press (2007). (In Chinese: 談允賢《女醫雜言》中醫古籍出版社)

Wu, Yi-Li, *Reproducing Women: Medicine, Metaphor, and Childbirth in Late Imperial China*; University of California Press (2010).

Zheng, Jin-Sheng, *Tan Yunxian, a woman physician of Ming dynasty, and her Nu yi za yan (Random talks of a woman physician)*; (article in Chinese); Chin J Med Hist, July 1999, Vol. 29, No. 3
http://wenku.baidu.com/view/8e7ddbcff61fb7360b4c65f1.html (accessed on 12/11/2014)
http://www.bufuzao.com/gushi/mingren/124130.html (same but text)

Zheng, Jin-Sheng, *Female Medical Workers in Ancient China; Current Perspectives in the History of Science in East Asia*, edited by Yung Sik Kim and Francesca Bray, 460-66. Seoul National University Press, 1999.
http://www.tcm-acupuncture.eu/Literatur/Fachartikel/englisch/female-medical-worker.htm (accessed on 12/9/2014)

Books about the general role of women in late imperial China:

Cass, Victoria B., *Dangerous Women: Warriors, Grannies, and Geishas of the Ming*; Rowman & Littlefield Publishers (1999).

Li, Wai-yee, *Women and National Trauma in Late Imperial Chinese Literature* (Harvard-Yenching Institute Monograph Series); Harvard University Asia Center (2014).

See, Lisa, *Peony in Love: A Novel*; Random House (2007).[1]

---

1. While this is a novel, it is well researched and can give the less academically minded reader an understanding of the lives of well off women at the time, and the emergence of women authors in the late *Ming* and early *Qīng* dynasties.

Books concerning or containing case studies in Chinese medicine

Furth, Charlotte, et al., editor, *Thinking with Cases: Specialist Knowledge in Chinese Cultural History*; University of Hawai'i Press (2007).

Grant, Joanna, *A Chinese Physician: Wang Ji and the 'Stone Mountain medical case histories'*; Routledgecurzon (2003).

Hsu, Elizabeth, *Pulse Diagnosis in Early Chinese Medicine: The Telling Touch*; University of Cambridge Press (2010).

Yang, Jizhou (author), Wilcox, Lorraine (translator), *The Great Compendium of Acupuncture and Moxibustion: Zhen Jiu Da Cheng, Volume 9,* The Chinese Medicine Database (2011).

Points

Liè Quē (LU 7)	列缺	45
Shǒu Sān Lǐ (LI 10)	手三里	63, 95
Qū Chí (LI 11)	曲池	45
Jiān Yú (LI 15)	肩寓	45
Chéng Mǎn (ST 20)	承滿	137
Qì Chōng (ST 30)	氣衝	119
Sān Lǐ (ST 36)	三里	74, 116
Pí Shù (UB 20)	脾腧	74, 116
Gāo Huāng (UB 43)	膏肓	74, 116
Jiān Shǐ (PC 5)	間使	63, 95
Nèi Guān (PC 6)	内關	63, 95
Zhī Gōu (SJ 6)	支溝	45
Tiān Jǐng (SJ 10)	天井	54, 63, 95
Yī Fēng (SJ 17)	醫風	54, 63, 67, 95
Jiān Jǐng (GB 21)	肩井	54, 63, 67, 95
Jué Gǔ (GB 39)	絕骨	95
Zhōng Jí (Rèn 3)	中極	119
Guān Yuán (Rèn 4)	關元	119
Qì Hǎi (Rèn 6)	氣海	119
Xià Wǎn (Rèn 10)	下脘	73, 76, 85, 113, 125
Zhōng Wǎn (Rèn 12)	中脘	73, 76, 85, 113, 125, 137
Shàng Wǎn (Rèn 13)	上脘	73, 76, 85, 113, 125
Dà Zhuì (Dū 14)	大椎	74, 116
Shí Guān (non-channel)	食關	76, 85, 113, 125
Xìng Lóng	興隆	126
Zhǒu Jiān (non-channel)	肘尖	54, 56, 95

Medicinals

dāng guī	當歸	43, 52, 61–62, 67–70, 82–83, 88–89, 99, 106–108, 110, 115, 118, 123, 132–133, 140
dāng guī shēn	當歸身	50
dāng guī wěi	當歸尾	65–66
dì gǔ pí	地骨皮	109
dì lóng	地龍	91
dìng fěn	定粉	124
dòng shù gēn	楝樹根	87
dú huó	獨活	72–73
dù zhòng	杜仲	47, 133
ē jiāo	阿膠	84
fáng fēng	防風	47, 87–89
fáng jǐ	防己	57, 59–60
fēi gǔ shēng fán	飛礬生礬	87
fěn shuāng	粉霜	124
fú líng	茯苓	43, 47, 61–62, 70, 78, 80–81, 83, 98, 101, 104–106, 110, 115–116, 123, 127, 130–131, 133, 140
fú shén	茯神	100, 128, 130
fù zǐ	附子	47
gān cǎo	甘草	43, 47, 50, 53, 59, 61–62, 65–66, 69–70, 72, 76, 81, 84, 89, 98, 101, 105–107, 111, 116–117, 127, 130, 141
gān sōng	甘松	112
gé gēn	葛根	50, 66
gǒu qǐ	枸杞	87, 133
gǒu qǐ gēn	枸杞根	108–109
guā lóu gēn	瓜蔞根	65–66
guǎng fang jǐ	廣防己	60
guǎng róng	廣茋	66
guī bǎn	龜板	44
hàn fang jǐ	漢防己	60
hǎo chá	好茶	90
hé shǒu wū	何首烏	111–112, 120–121
hé yè	荷葉	39, 41, 88, 101, 128
hēi qiān niú	黑牽牛	135
hòu pǔ	厚朴	79, 81–83, 127
huá shí	滑石	89
huáng bǎi	黃柏	44, 47, 59, 66, 91
huáng dān	黃丹	91
huáng jīng	黃荊	87
huáng lián	黃連	39, 42, 66, 80, 83–84, 103, 106–107, 129–130
huáng qí	黃耆	50, 117, 133

160

162

Formula Index

General Index

166

The Chinese Medicine Database

www.cm-db.com

The Chinese Medicine Database has been organized around one central principle -- translation of Classical Asian texts, and dissemination of that information.

There are thousands of Asian medicine texts that have never been translated. We have compiled a small list on our website of the ones that we have found, but we believe that there are tens of thousands of documents that span from the *Hàn* Dynasty to pre-Republican times. Most of these documents will never be read by people in the West, simply because of lack of translation.

We have created a vehicle, that allows interested practitioners, students, institutions, and scholars to help support and fund the translation of these documents, and then mine and synthesize the data that is gained from these texts.

The Database contains:

Monographs on:
690 Single Herbs
1510 Formulas
Mayway's Patents
ITM's Formulations
Golden Flowers Formulations
Classical Pearls Formulations by Heiner Fruehauf
OBGYN Modifications to Formulas
Single Points: the 361 Regular Points
Time Line of the History of Chinese Medicine

Beer Hall Lecture Series
Watch videos from our monthly Beer Hall lecture series with guest speakers such as: Arnaud Versluys, Subhuti Dharmananda, Jason Robertson, Craig Mitchell, Michael Max, Lorraine Wilcox, and Ed Neal.

Play STORT
Play our free online game STORT where you can learn Chinese while having a bit of fun (www.cm-db.com/stort).

15,000 Western Diagnoses with ICD-9 Codes

A Chinese-English dictionary:
Containing over 102,943 terms, including the Eastland and the WHO term sets.

A Western Book search containing:
Fenner's Complete Formulary
   by B. Fenner
The 1918 Dispensatory of the United States of America
   Edited by Joseph P. Remington, Horatio C. Woods and others
The Eclectic Materia Medica, Pharmacology and Therapeutics
   by Harvey Wickes Felter, M.D.

A Personal Dashboard, which allows users to:
Blog
Take notes on any monograph.
Search for other users by city, state, country and name.
Make friends all around the world.
Share and compare notes with friends.
Personalize your dashboard by adding photos, and information about your practice.

Translations:

Shāng Hán Lái Sū Jí	傷寒來蘇集	Renewal of Treatise on Cold Damage
Qí Jīng Bā Mài Kǎo	奇經八脈考	Explanation of the Eight Vessels of the Marvellous Meridians
Shāng Hán Míng Lǐ Lùn	傷寒明理論	Treatise on Enlightening the Principles of Cold Damage
Wú Jū Tōng Yī Àn	吳鞠通医案	Case Studies of Wú Jūtōng
The Nàn Jīng	難經	The Classic of Difficulties
The Zàng Fǔ Biāo Běn Hán Rè Xū Shí Yòng Yào Shì	臟腑標本寒熱虛實用藥式	Viscera and Bowels, Tip and Root, Cold and Heat, Vacuity and Repletion Model for Using Medicinals
Wēn Rè Lún	温熱論	Treatise on Warm Heat Disease
Shāng Hán Shé Jiàn	傷寒舌鑒	Tongue Mirror of Cold Damage
Xǔ Shì Yī Àn	許氏醫案	Case Histories of Master Xǔ
Fǔ Xìng Jué Zàng Fǔ Yòng Yào Fǎ Yào	輔行決臟腑用藥法要	Secret Instructions for Assisting the Body: Essential Methods for the Application of Drugs to the Viscera & Bowels
Biāo Yōu Fù	標幽賦	Indicating the Obscure

Liú Juān Zǐ Guǐ Yí Fāng	劉涓子鬼遺方	Liu Juanzi's Formulas Inherited from Ghosts
Shèn Jí Chú Yán	慎疾芻言	Precautions in Illness: My Humble Thoughts
Yào Zhèng Jì Yí	藥症忌宜	Medicinals & Patterns Contraindications & Appropriate [Choices]
Fù Kē Wèn Dá	婦科問答	Questions and Answers in Gynecology
Nèi Jīng Zhī Yào	內經知要	Essential Knowledge from the Nèijīng
Běn Cǎo Bèi Yào	本草備要	The Essential Completion of Traditional Materia Medica
Bǎi Zhèng Fù（Jù Yīng）	百症賦《聚英》	Ode of the Hundred Diseases from The Great Compendium of Acupuncture-Moxibustion

Benefits:

Subscribers to the Database receive a 10% discount on our published books when they are in pre-release.

We translate texts as often, and in quantities that reflect our user base. The larger amount of subscribers that we have, the more translation that we can accomplish.

Published Books:

2008 Bèi Jí Qiān Jīn Yào Fāng 備急千金要方:
Essential Prescriptions Worth a Thousand Gold Pieces
For Emergencies. vol. 2-4
by Sūn Sīmiǎo 孫思邈
Translated by Sabine Wilms.
ISBN 978-0-9799552-0-4
Out of Print

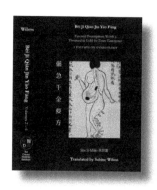

2010 Zhēn Jiǔ Dà Chéng 針灸大成:
The Great Compendium of Acupuncture & Moxibustion vol. I
by Yáng Jìzhōu 楊繼洲
Translated by Sabine Wilms.
ISBN 978-0-9799552-2-8

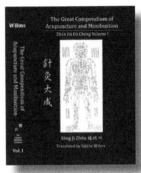

2010 Zhēn Jiǔ Dà Chéng 針灸大成:
The Great Compendium of Acupuncture & Moxibustion vol. V
by Yáng Jìzhōu 楊繼洲
Translated by Lorraine Wilcox.
ISBN 978-0-9799552-4-2

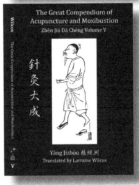

2010 Jīn Guì Fāng Gē Kuò 金匱方歌括:
Formulas from the Golden Cabinet with Songs vol. I - III
by Chén Xiūyuán 陳修園
Translated by Sabine Wilms.
ISBN 978-0-9799552-5-9

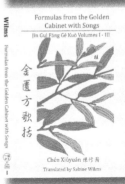

2011 Zhēn Jiǔ Dà Chéng 針灸大成:
The Great Compendium of Acupuncture & Moxibustion vol. VIII
by Yáng Jìzhōu 楊繼洲
Translated by Yue Lu.
ISBN 978-0-9799552-7-3

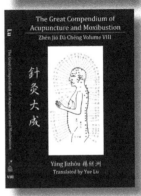

2011 Zhēn Jiǔ Dà Chéng 針灸大成:
The Great Compendium of Acupuncture & Moxibustion vol. IX
by Yáng Jìzhōu 楊繼洲
Translated by Lorraine Wilcox.
ISBN 978-0-9799552-6-6

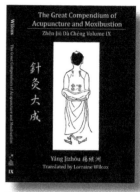

2012 Raising the Dead and Returning Life: Emergency Medicine of the Qīng Dynasty
by Bào Xiāng'áo 鮑相璈
Translated by Lorraine Wilcox.
ISBN 978-0-9799552-3-5

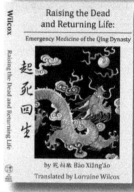

2014 Zhēn Jiǔ Zī Shēng Jīng 針灸資生經:
The Classic of Supporting Life with Acupuncture and Moxibustion Vol. I-III
by Wáng Zhízhōng 王執中
Translated by Yue Lu.
ISBN 978-0-9799552-1-1

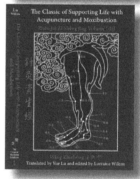

2014 Jīn Guì Fāng Gē Kuò 金匱方歌括:
Formulas from the Golden Cabinet with Songs
vol. IV - VI
by Chén Xiūyuán 陳修園
Translated by Eran Even.
ISBN 978-0-9799552-8-0

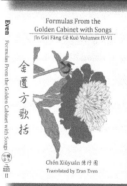

174

2015 Zhēn Jiǔ Zī Shēng Jīng 針灸資生經:
The Classic of Supporting Life with Acupuncture and
Moxibustion Vol. IV-VII
by Wáng Zhízhōng 王執中
Translated by Yue Lu.
ISBN 978-0-9799552-9-7

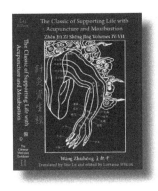

Printed in the USA
CPSIA information can be obtained
at www.ICGtesting.com
LVHW070208130923
758063LV00007B/165